Copyright

Copyright © [2023] by Taylor Johnson

Disclaimer

The content presented in this book is intended solely for educational and informational purposes. The author and publisher of this Book are not medical professionals, and the content should not be considered a substitute for professional medical advice, diagnosis, or treatment. Whenever you have inquiries concerning your health or medical condition, make sure to consult a qualified healthcare provider for advice.

The recipes, tips, and suggestions presented in this Book are based on the author's personal experiences, research, and knowledge in the field of nutrition and wellness. However, individual results may vary, and it is important to listen to your body and make choices that align with your specific needs and circumstances. It is recommended to consult with a healthcare professional or a registered dietitian before making any significant changes to your diet or lifestyle.

The author and publisher do not assume any responsibility or liability for any loss, injury, or damage incurred as a result of the use or reliance upon the information provided in this Book. The reader assumes full responsibility for any actions taken based on the content of this Book.

Furthermore, the mention of specific products, brands, or organizations in this Book is for informational purposes only and does not imply endorsement or affiliation. The author and publisher do not have any financial or professional relationships with these entities unless explicitly stated.

While every effort has been made to ensure the accuracy and reliability of the information provided, the author and publisher do not guarantee the completeness, timeliness, or accuracy of the content. They disclaim any responsibility for any errors or omissions.

By reading and utilizing the information in this Book, you agree to do so at your own risk. The author and publisher shall not be held responsible for any consequences or adverse effects that may arise from the use of the information contained in this Book.

Thank you for understanding and acknowledging the disclaimer. Always prioritize your health and consult with a qualified professional for personalized advice and guidance.

Table of Content

Introduction

Are you ready to embark on a flavorful journey that will transform your mornings and revitalize your body? Look no further! Introducing The 7-Day Smoothie Challenge: How to unleash the Power of Everyday Smoothies! This groundbreaking Book is here to guide you on a delicious adventure, helping you discover the wonders of everyday smoothies in just one week.

In a world filled with complicated recipes and overwhelming ingredient lists, we understand the desire for simplicity without compromising on taste. That's why we've designed this 7-day challenge, tailored specifically for you. Say goodbye to breakfast monotony and hello to a vibrant and energizing start to your day.

Chapter by chapter, you'll explore the endless possibilities of everyday smoothies:

Delightful concoctions that tantalize your taste buds

Power-packed with essential nutrients for your body

Suitable for both seasoned smoothie enthusiasts and beginners

Packed with all the information needed to become a smoothie maestro

Introduction

Why should you incorporate smoothies into your daily routine? The benefits are truly remarkable. From increased energy levels and improved digestion to glowing skin and boosted immunity, everyday smoothies are the secret to a healthier and happier you.

In The 7-Day Smoothie Challenge, we go beyond the basics. We equip you with:

The essential tools

Knowledge

Mouthwatering recipes

To turn your kitchen into a smoothie paradise. From luscious apple blends to tropical banana creations, each day of the challenge offers a unique and delightful experience. We'll explore the harmonious fusion of flavors, unlocking the secrets behind perfect pairings like strawberries and bananas, apples and pears, and oranges and lemons.

But this challenge is more than just a collection of recipes. It's an invitation to unleash your creativity. We encourage you to:

Experiment with different ingredients

Tailor the recipes to your flavor preferences

Create your own signature smoothie masterpieces

We'll provide you with variations and suggestions along the way, ensuring that every sip is a celebration of your unique palate.

Introduction

So, are you ready to embrace:

The sweet
The savory
The delicious

world of everyday smoothies?

Join us on this 7-day adventure and witness the incredible transformation that awaits.

Get your blender ready!
Stock up on fresh produce!
Prepare to embark!

This journey will invigorate your mornings and nourish your body from within. So, let's dive into "The 7-Day Smoothie Challenge" and discover How to Unleash the Power of Everyday Smoothies! Let's:

Blend
Sip
Savor

Our way to a healthier and happier you!

THE 7-DAY

SMOOTHIE

CHALLENGE

HOW TO UNLEASH THE POWER OF EVERYDAY SMOOTHIES!

Taylor Johnson

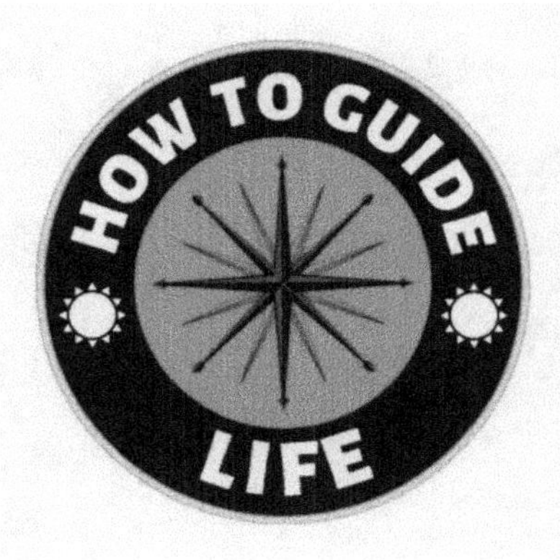

Chapter 1: Why Everyday Smoothies?

Welcome to the vibrant world of everyday smoothies! This chapter explores numerous reasons adding smoothies into your daily routine can result in significant changes to your health and well-being. Get ready to discover the extraordinary benefits that await you as you embark on this delicious journey.

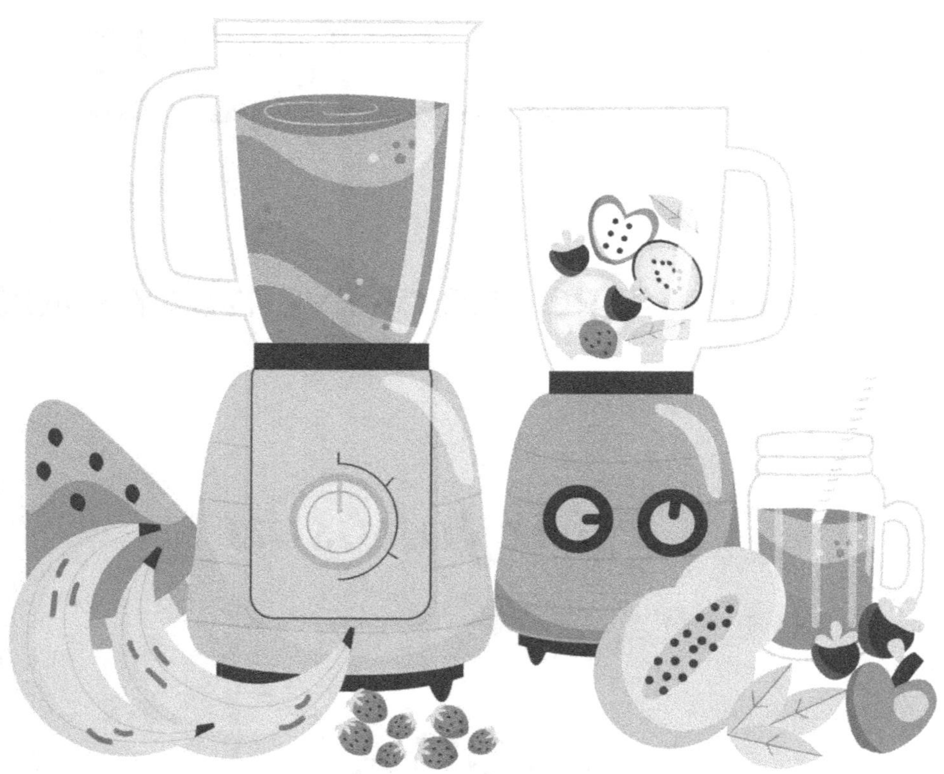

Chapter 1: Why Everyday Smoothies?

Section 1: Fuel Your Body with Natural Energy

Picture this: It's early morning, and instead of reaching for that caffeine fix or a sugar-loaded breakfast, you indulge in a vibrant, nutrient-rich smoothie. One sip, and you can feel your body awakening, energized by the natural goodness within. Everyday smoothies offer a sustainable and long-lasting source of energy, fueled by the powerful combination of:

Fruits

Vegetables

Other Wholesome Ingredients

Say goodbye to mid-morning slumps and hello to sustained vitality throughout the day.

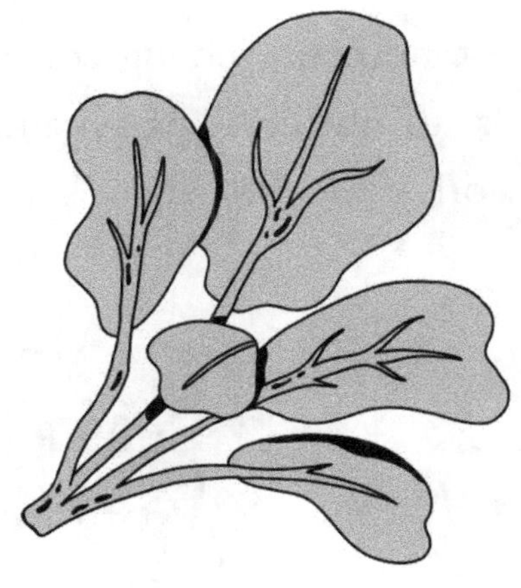

Chapter 1: Why Everyday Smoothies?

1.1 The Power of Nutrient-Rich Ingredients

At the heart of everyday smoothies are the ingredients that fuel your body with natural energy. Fruits like bananas, berries, and citrus fruits provide a burst of natural sugars and essential vitamins. They deliver the sweetness you crave without the crash that comes from processed sugars.

Meanwhile, leafy greens such as:

Spinach
Kale
Swiss chard

Pack a punch of nutrients like:

Iron
Calcium
Antioxidants

Including these nutrient-rich ingredients into your smoothies, provides your body with the fuel it needs to thrive. The vitamins, minerals, and antioxidants present in these ingredients work synergistically to support:

Immune System
Enhance cognitive function
Promote overall welll-being

Chapter 1: Why Everyday Smoothies?

1.2 Balancing Macronutrients for Sustained Energy

To achieve sustained energy throughout the day, it's important to strike a balance between macronutrients in your smoothies. For maintaining stable blood sugar levels and lasting source of energy

Protein
Healthy fats
Complex carbohydrates

Play key roles.

Protein, found in ingredients like:

Greek yogurt
Nut butter
Plant-based protein powders

Helps to keep you full and satisfied, while supporting muscle growth and repair.

Healthy fats, such as:

Avocados
Nuts
Seeds

Provide a slow burning source of energy and aid in the absorption of fat-soluble vitamins.

Complex carbohydrates, such as oats, quinoa, or sweet potatoes, provide a steady release of glucose, preventing energy crashes and keeping you fueled for longer.

Chapter 1: Why Everyday Smoothies?
1.2 Balancing Macronutrients for Sustained Energy

By incorporating these macronutrients into your smoothies, you:

Create a balanced and nourishing blend

Helps maintain your energy levels throughout the day

Say goodbye to the dreaded 3 PM slump

Say hello to a steady stream of natural energy

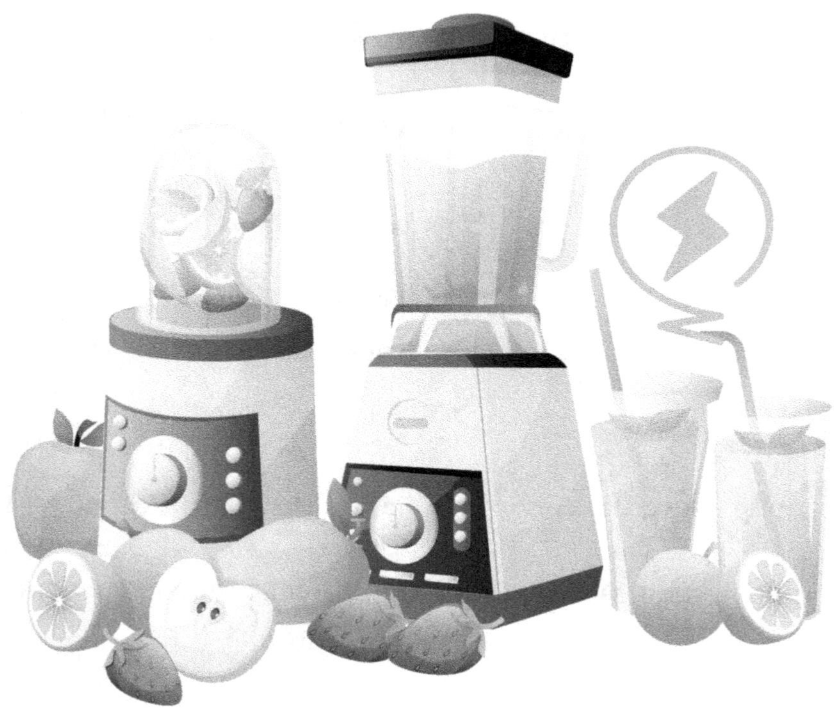

Chapter 1: Why Everyday Smoothies?

1.3 Hydration for Optimal Energy

Maintaining adequate hydration is crucial for sustaining energy levels and promoting overall well-being. Smoothies can be an excellent way to stay hydrated, especially when you use hydrating bases like coconut water, herbal teas, or even plain water as the liquid component of your blend.

Hydration plays a crucial role in maintaining optimal bodily function, it aids in numerous ways such as:

Regulating body temperature
Digestion
Nutrient absorption

When you incorporate hydrating bases into your smoothies, you are enhancing the flavor and also replenishing your body's fluids.

Imagine sipping on a:

Refreshing watermelon smoothie
Refreshing cucumber smoothie

Made with ingredients that helps to:

Hydrate your body
Quench your thirst
Provides you with natural energy boost

With every sip, you're replenishing your body and invigorating your senses, ready to tackle whatever the day brings.

Chapter 1: Why Everyday Smoothies?

1.4 Harnessing the Power of Natural Antioxidants

Antioxidants are superheroes when it comes to fueling your body with natural energy.

These powerful compounds fight against:

Damaging effects of free radicals

Oxidative stress

Cell damage

This can result in tiredness and reduced energy levels

Fruits and vegetables are abundant sources of antioxidants, ranking among the highest are:

Berries

Cherries

Dark leafy greens

By incorporating these antioxidant-rich ingredients into your smoothies, you're:

Providing your body with protective shield against oxidative damage

Supporting your energy levels

Improving your overall well-being

Imagine enjoying a delicious blueberry and spinach smoothie, bursting with antioxidants that promote energy production and cellular health. With every sip, you're nourishing your body from the inside out, unlocking a vibrant energy that lasts throughout the day.

Chapter 1: Why Everyday Smoothies?

1.5 A Wholesome Approach to Fueling Your Body

Everyday smoothies offer a wholesome approach to fueling your body with natural energy. They provide a very convenient and also delicious way to add various nutrient-dense ingredients into your diet.

By embracing the power of everyday smoothies, you're:

Providing your body with the vital nutrients it requires to thrive

Enhancing your vitality

Unlocking your full potential

Say goodbye to the roller coaster of energy crashes and hello to a sustained, vibrant energy that fuels your every endeavor. With every sip of your nutrient-packed and delicious smoothie, you're making a mindful choice to put first your health and well-being.

So, are you ready to embark on a journey towards sustained energy and vitality? Let The 7-Day Smoothie Challenge: How to Unleash the Power of Everyday Smoothies! be your guide as we explore mouthwatering recipes, expert tips, and a wealth of knowledge to help you fuel your body with natural energy. Get your blender ready, and let's begin this incredible adventure together!

Chapter 1: Why Everyday Smoothies?

Section 2: Amplify Your Nutrient Intake

Do you struggle to consume enough fruits and vegetables? You're not alone. Many people find it challenging to meet their daily recommended intake of essential nutrients. However, with everyday smoothies, you can effortlessly boost your nutrient intake in a delicious and convenient way.

These blended delights are packed with:

Vitamins

Minerals

Antioxidants

Fiber

Providing a concentrated dose of nourishment for your body. Experience the joy of effortlessly meeting your nutritional needs with every sip.

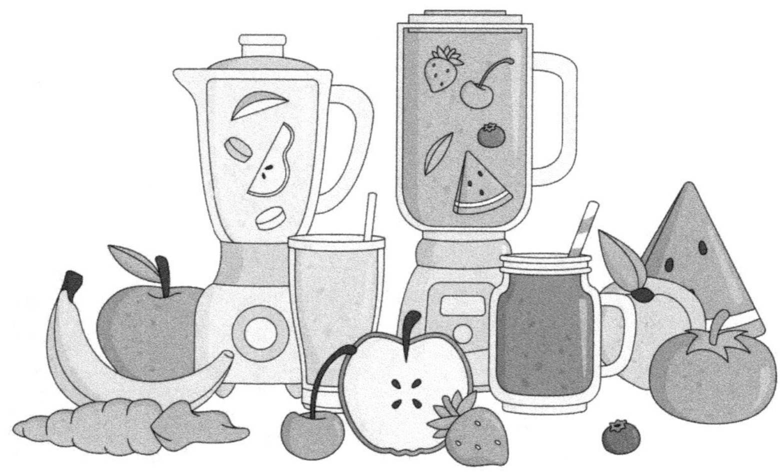

Chapter 1: Why Everyday Smoothies?

2.1 The Nutritional Powerhouse of Fruits and Vegetables

Fruits and vegetables are nature's nutritional powerhouses. They overflow with a diverse range of indispensable vitamins, minerals, and antioxidants. However, incorporating the recommended servings into your daily diet can be a daunting task. That's where everyday smoothies come to the rescue.

By blending fruits and vegetables into a smoothie, you can without much effort consume a variety of these nutrient rich foods in one delicious drink.

Imagine savoring a refreshing green smoothie packed with leafy greens like:

Kale
Spinach
Cucumber

Along with juicy fruits like:

Pineapple
Mango
Kiwi

With every sip, you're flooding your body with a host of vital nutrients and an abundance of vitamins:

A
C
K

Chapter 1: Why Everyday Smoothies?

2.2 Unlocking the Nutritional Potential

The blending process breaks down the cell walls of fruits and vegetables, making their nutrients more readily absorbed by the body. This means that when you enjoy a smoothie, you're maximizing the nutritional potential of the ingredients, ensuring that your body can fully benefit from their goodness.

For example, the powerful antioxidant lycopene found in tomatoes becomes more bioavailable when blended, promoting heart health and reducing the risk of chronic diseases. Similarly, the soluble fiber in fruits and vegetables:

Are more accessible to the digestive system

Support healthy digestion

Aid in nutrient absorption

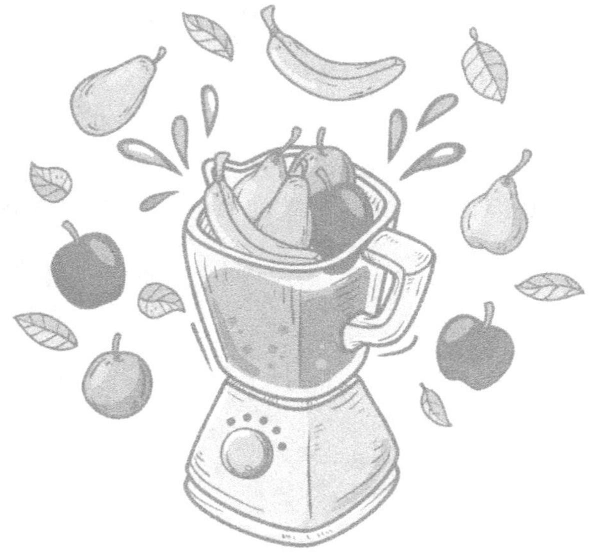

Chapter 1: Why Everyday Smoothies?

2.3 Fiber: The Unsung Hero

Including fiber in a healthy diet is essential:

> **It supports digestive health**
>
> **Regulates blood sugar levels**
>
> **Promotes a feeling of fullness.**

Unfortunately, many people fall short of meeting their daily fiber needs. But fear not, because everyday smoothies can come to the rescue.

When you blend whole fruits and vegetables, you retain their fiber content, providing a satisfying dose of this essential nutrient. Fiber helps slow down digestion, preventing blood sugar spikes and crashes, and keeping you feeling satiated for longer. With every sip of your fiber-rich smoothie, you're nourishing your body and supporting optimal digestive function.

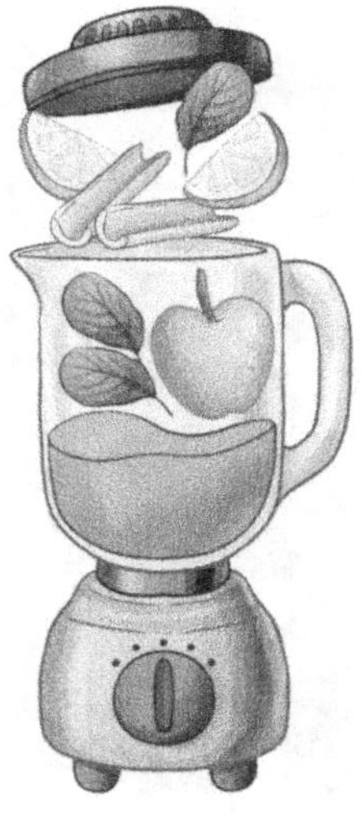

Chapter 1: Why Everyday Smoothies?

2.4 Antioxidants for Optimal Health

Antioxidants are your body's defenders against free radicals. Free radicals are harmful molecules that can cause cellular damage and contribute to chronic diseases.

Fruits and vegetables are packed with:

Antioxidants

Vitamins C, E

Various plant compounds like flavonoids and carotenoids

When you enjoy everyday smoothies, you're flooding your body with a wealth of antioxidants, promoting optimal health and well-being. From the vibrant purple of blueberries to the rich orange of carrots, each ingredient brings its unique antioxidant profile, protecting your cells and supporting overall vitality.

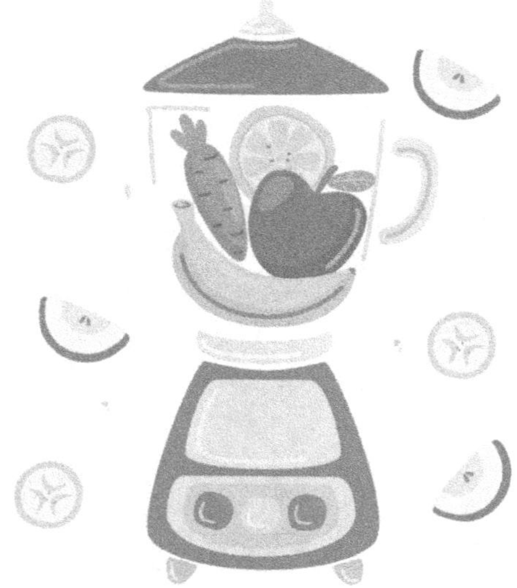

Chapter 1: Why Everyday Smoothies?

2.5 Supercharging with Superfoods

Superfoods are nutrient-dense ingredients known for their exceptional health benefits.

Some examples are:

Chia seeds

Spirulina

Matcha powder

These powerhouse ingredients can take your everyday smoothies to the next level.

Incorporating superfoods into your smoothies allows you to amplify the nutritional density of your blends. Imagine adding a tablespoon of flaxseed for a boost of omega-3 fatty acids or a teaspoon of maca powder for hormone balance and increased energy. With each spoonful of these superfoods, you're elevating your nutrient intake and experiencing the benefits of these extraordinary ingredients.

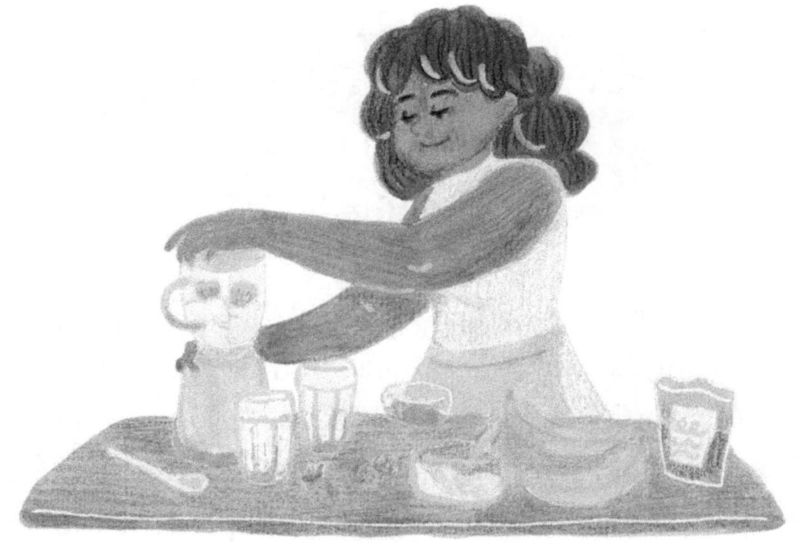

Chapter 1: Why Everyday Smoothies?

2.6 Tailoring Smoothies to Meet Your Nutritional Needs

One of the remarkable aspects of everyday smoothies is their versatility. You have the freedom to customize your blends to meet your unique nutritional needs.

Whether you're:

Focusing on specific vitamins or minerals
Aiming for a higher protein content
Following a particular dietary pattern

Your smoothie can be tailored to align with your goals.

Experiment with different combinations, explore new ingredients, and listen to your body's cravings. By fine tuning your smoothies to meet your nutritional needs, you'll experience the joy of providing your body with the specific nourishment it requires.

Section 2: Amplify Your Nutrient Intake takes you on a journey through the nutritional power of everyday smoothies.

By blending:

Fruits
Vegetables
Superfoods

You're elevating your nutrient intake and nourishing your body from within. Get ready to discover a world of vibrant flavors, concentrated nutrition, and the incredible benefits of effortlessly meeting your nutritional needs. Let "The 7-Day Smoothie Challenge: How to Unleash the Power of Everyday Smoothies!" be your guide to unlocking the full potential of these nutritional powerhouses and embracing a healthier, more vibrant lifestyle.

Chapter 1: Why Everyday Smoothies?

Section 3: Aid Digestion and Promote Gut Health

If you've ever experienced:

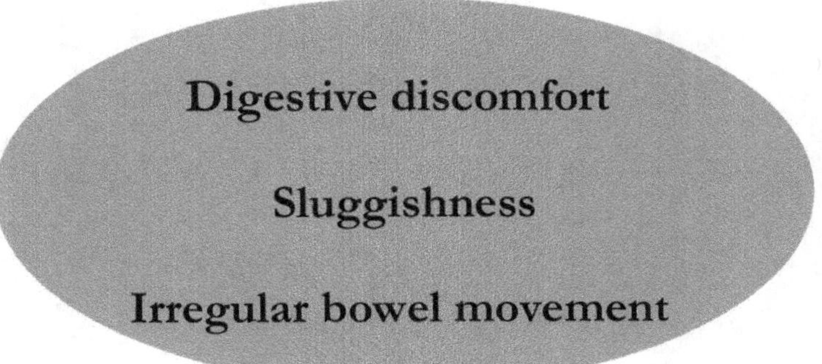

You may know how important it is to support your gut health. Everyday smoothies are a fantastic tool to aid digestion and promote a healthy gut. The natural fibers present in fruits and vegetables help regulate bowel movements and maintain a healthy digestive system. Additionally, certain ingredients, such as ginger or yogurt, can further support digestion and soothe any tummy troubles you may have. Get ready to say goodbye to digestive woes and embrace a happier, more balanced gut.

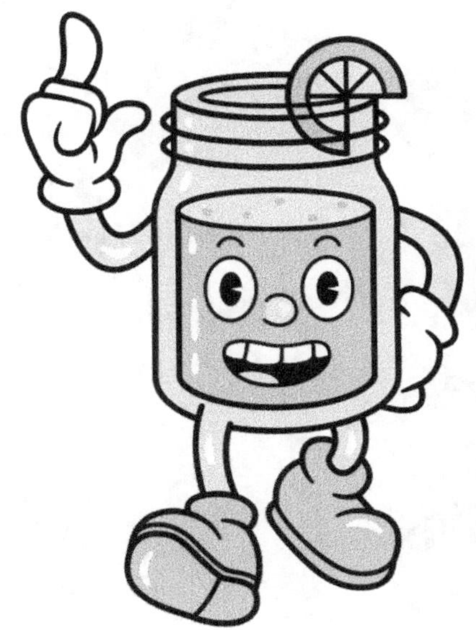

Chapter 1: Why Everyday Smoothies?
3.1 The Power of Fiber for Digestive Health

Fiber is the overlooked hero when it comes to maintaining a healthy digestive system.

It adds bulk to your stool

Facilitating regular bowel movements

Preventing constipation

Fruits and vegetables are wonderful sources of fiber. When incorporated into everyday smoothies, they can significantly contribute to your daily fiber intake.

With each sip of your fiber-rich smoothie, you're nourishing your gut microbiota. Gut microbiotas are the trillions of beneficial bacteria that reside in your digestive tract. These friendly microbes thrive on fiber, fermenting it into short-chain fatty acids that support gut health and promote a balanced digestive environment.

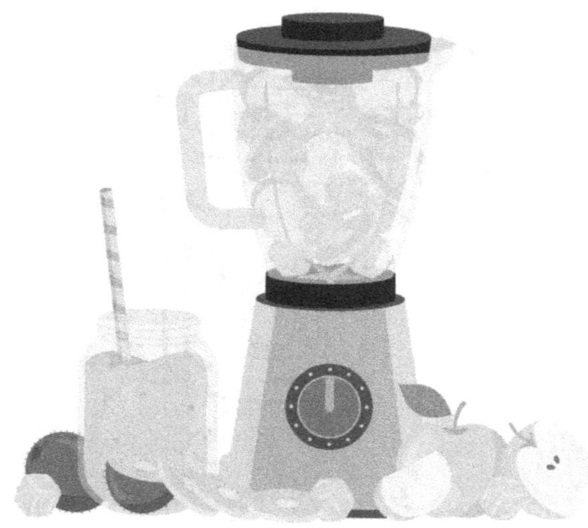

Chapter 1: Why Everyday Smoothies?

3.2 Ginger: The Digestive Soother

For centuries, ginger has been employed to support digestion and relieve gastrointestinal discomfort. Its natural compounds, such as gingerol, have powerful anti-inflammatory and soothing properties. By incorporating ginger into your smoothies, you can harness its digestive benefits and promote a calm, happy tummy.

Whether it's a dash of fresh ginger root or a sprinkle of ground ginger powder, this humble spice can work wonders for your digestive system.

It can help:

Alleviate nausea

Reduce bloating

Ease stomach cramps.

So, if you're looking to support digestion and add a touch of warmth and zest to your smoothies, don't forget to invite ginger to the party.

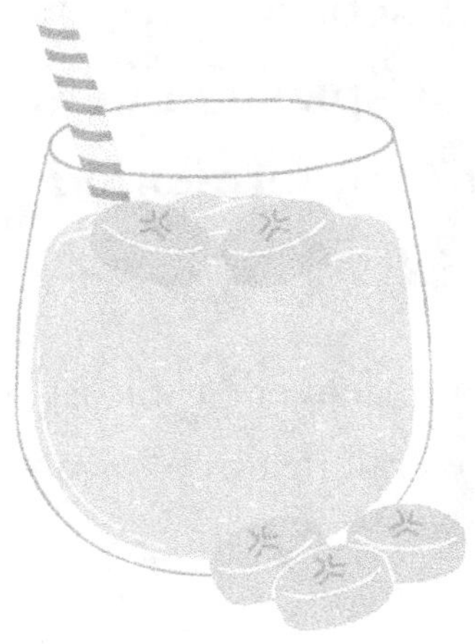

Chapter 1: Why Everyday Smoothies?

3.3 Probiotics: Cultivate a Healthy Gut Microbiome

Your gut microbiome, the community of microorganisms living in your intestines, plays a crucial role in:

Digestion

Metabolism

Overall health

Probiotics, which are useful bacteria and can help maintain a balanced gut microbiome.

They are found in foods like:

Yogurt

Kefir

Fermented vegetables

Including probiotic-rich ingredients in your smoothies can introduce these beneficial bacteria into your digestive system, promoting a healthy gut flora.

Whether you opt for:

A scoop of yogurt

A splash of kefir

A spoon full of fermented vegetables

Incorporating these additions can deliver a boost of probiotics, promoting better digestion and contributing to the overall health of your gut.

Chapter 1: Why Everyday Smoothies?

3.4 Soothing Smoothie Blends for Digestive Comfort

Sometimes, our digestive system needs a little extra love and care. Smoothies can be a gentle and soothing way to support digestive comfort, especially when you incorporate ingredients known for their soothing properties.

For example:

Mint leaves have a cooling effect on the digestive system and can help relieve indigestion or stomach discomfort.

Aloe vera can have a soothing effect on the gut lining, reducing inflammation and promoting healing. When consumed in its edible form

Ginger can aid in digestion by reducing bloating and soothing an upset stomach

Blending these soothing ingredients with fruits and vegetables can create smoothies that nourish your body and provide relief to your digestive system.

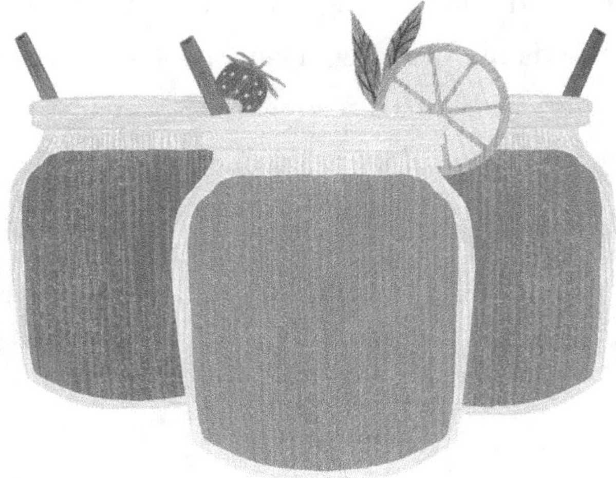

Chapter 1: Why Everyday Smoothies?

3.5 Mindful Eating for Better Digestion

In addition to the ingredients you choose for your smoothies, practicing mindful eating can also contribute to better digestion.

Take the time to savor each sip of your smoothie, paying attention to the:

Flavors

Textures

Sensations in your body

Chew your smoothie if it contains fibrous ingredients to aid the digestive process.

By adopting mindful eating practices, you allow your body to fully process and absorb the nutrients from your smoothie. This mindful approach to eating can further aid in stress reduction, given the intricate connection between digestion and emotional well-being.

Section 3: Aid Digestion and Promote Gut Health reminds us of the vital role our digestive system plays in overall well-being. With everyday smoothies, you have the power to support your gut health and alleviate digestive discomfort. From fiber-rich fruits and vegetables to soothing ingredients like ginger and probiotics, each sip of your smoothie can contribute to a happier, more balanced gut. Get ready to nourish your digestive system and experience the joy of a healthier, happier you.

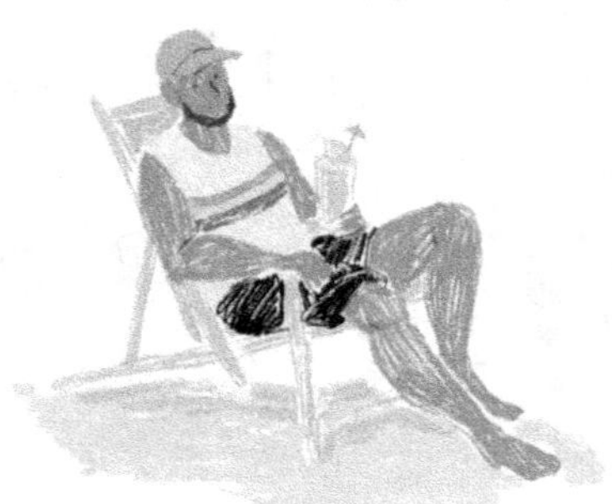

Chapter 1: Why Everyday Smoothies?

Section 4: Enhance Weight Management and Satiety

Many individuals have a regular goal to maintain a healthy weight. With everyday smoothies, you have a powerful ally in your weight management journey. These nutrient-rich blends can help you stay full for extended periods, decreasing the chances of indulging in unhealthy snacks or overeating. By incorporating a balance of fruits, vegetables, and protein sources into your smoothies, you can optimize satiety and support your weight management goals. Discover the secret to feeling satisfied and nourished while achieving a healthier body composition.

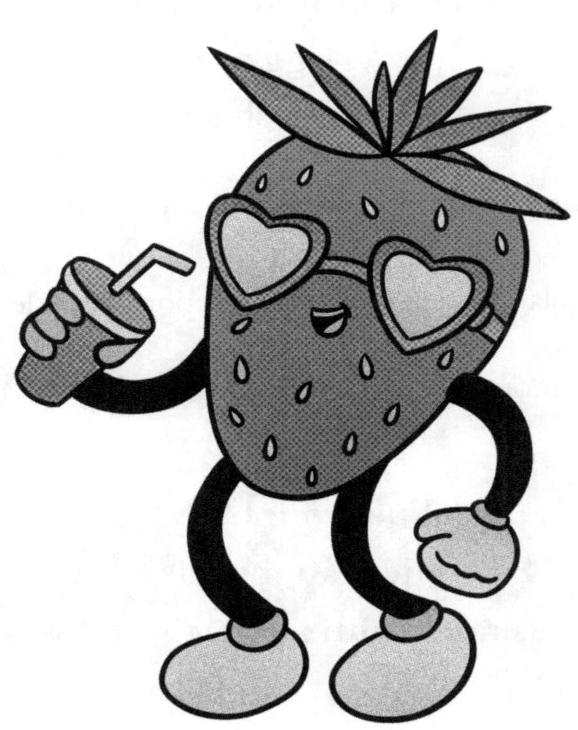

Chapter 1: Why Everyday Smoothies?

4.1 The Satiating Power of Protein

Protein, a vital macronutrient, plays a fundamental role in managing weight effectively. Including protein in your smoothies can promote feelings of fullness and help curb cravings throughout the day. Whether you choose plant-based proteins like:

Tofu
Greek yogurt
Almond butter

Or opt for animal-based options like:

Whey protein powder
Eggs
Cottage cheese

Incorporating protein into your smoothies can make a significant difference.

Protein not only helps regulate appetite but also supports muscle maintenance and repair.

By including an adequate amount of protein in your smoothies, you can:

Fuel your body
Promote lean muscle mass
Improve overall health and weight management

Chapter 1: Why Everyday Smoothies?

4.2 Fiber: The Satiety Superstar

Fiber is another key component that enhances satiety and supports weight management. Fruits and vegetables are excellent sources of dietary fiber, when blended into smoothies, they provide a concentrated dose of this satiating nutrient.

Fiber takes longer to digest, keeping you feeling satisfied for longer periods. It also adds bulk to your smoothies, creating a more substantial and fulfilling texture. By including fiber-rich ingredients such as:

leafy greens

Chia seeds

Flaxseeds

In your smoothies, you can promote a feeling of fullness and support your weight management efforts.

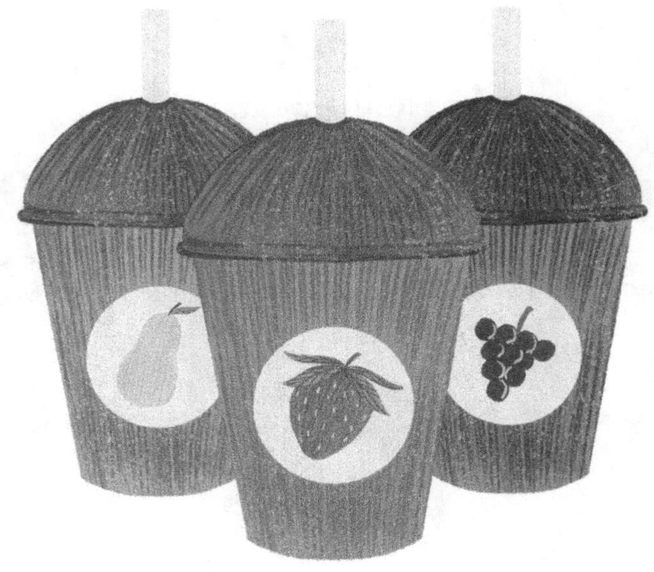

Chapter 1: Why Everyday Smoothies?

4.3 Balancing Macros for Optimal Satiety

Achieving a balance of macronutrients in your smoothies is key to enhancing satiety. While protein and fiber play vital roles, don't overlook the importance of incorporating healthy fats and complex carbohydrates into your blends.

Healthy fats, such as:

Avocado

Nut butters

Coconut milk

Provide a rich and creamy texture to your smoothies while contributing to feelings of fullness. Complex carbohydrates, found in ingredients like oats or quinoa, release energy slowly, helping to maintain stable blood sugar levels and prevent energy crashes.

By including a combination of:

Protein

Fiber

Healthy fats

Complex carbohydrates

In your smoothies, you create a well-rounded blend that satisfies your taste buds and your hunger.

Chapter 1: Why Everyday Smoothies?

4.4 Mindful Portions and Enjoyment

While smoothies can be an excellent tool for weight management, it's essential to practice mindful portions and mindful eating. Although smoothies are nutritious, they still contribute to your overall calorie intake. Be mindful of the ingredients and portion sizes to align with your specific goals.

Additionally, take the time to fully enjoy and savor each sip of your smoothie.

Sit down

Relax

Be present

With your beverage.

By slowing down and savoring the flavors and textures, you can enhance the overall satisfaction and enjoyment of your smoothie experience.

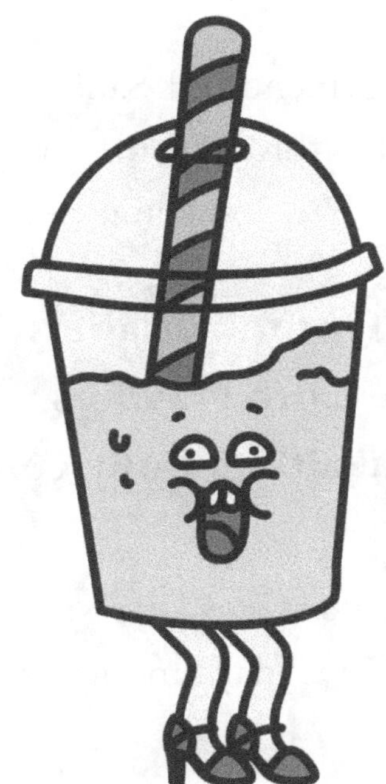

Chapter 1: Why Everyday Smoothies?

4.5 Long-Term Success with Everyday Smoothies

Incorporating everyday smoothies into your weight management journey can offer long-term success and sustainable results. By prioritizing nutrient-dense ingredients, balancing macros, and practicing mindful eating, you can harness the power of smoothies to support your weight management goals.

Remember, the key to success is:

Consistency
Discovering a personalized routine that suits your needs
Maintaining a balanced and varied ingredient selection

Experiment with different flavors, ingredients, and combinations to keep your smoothie experience exciting and enjoyable. With dedication and a commitment to nourishing your body, everyday smoothies can be a delicious and effective tool in achieving your weight management aspirations.

Section 4: Enhance Weight Management and Satiety empowers you to take control of your weight management journey through the power of everyday smoothies. By incorporating protein, fiber, healthy fats, and complex carbohydrates, you can:

Optimize satiety
Curb cravings
Support a healthier body composition

Get ready to feel satisfied, nourished, and one step closer to achieving your weight management goals with "Delicious Everyday Smoothies."

Chapter 1: Why Everyday Smoothies?

Section 5: Radiant Skin and Natural Detoxification

Your skin is a reflection of your internal health, and everyday smoothies can contribute to a glowing complexion. The abundance of antioxidants found in:

Fruits

Vegetables

Nuts

Assists in countering free radicals, which can lead to premature aging and skin damage. Additionally, certain ingredients like berries or leafy greens support natural detoxification processes, promoting clear and radiant skin from the inside out. Say hello to a youthful glow and revel in the beauty-boosting benefits of everyday smoothies.

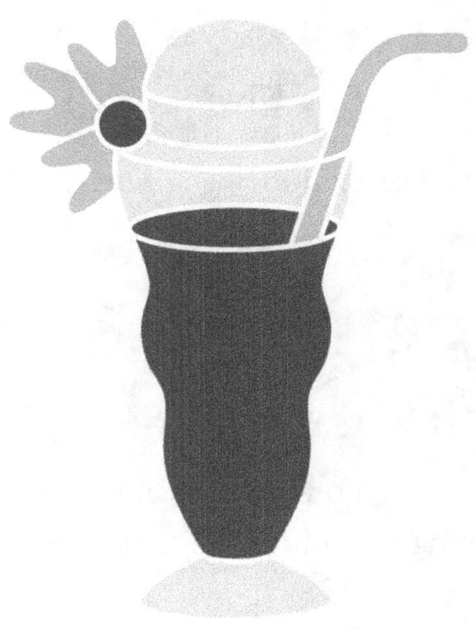

Chapter 1: Why Everyday Smoothies?

5.1 Antioxidants: The Skin's Best Friend

Unstable molecules known as free radicals can harm your skin cells and accelerate the aging process prematurely. The great news is antioxidants can effectively neutralize these damaging molecules, safeguarding your skin against oxidative stress.

Everyday smoothies provide a convenient and delicious way to flood your body with a wide range of antioxidants.

Some colorful fruits rich in antioxidants such as vitamin C and beta-carotene are:

Berries

Citrus fruits

Pineapples

Some tropical delights rich in antioxidants such as vitamin C and beta-carotene are:

Mangoes

Papayas

Kiwis

Some Leafy greens also packed with skin-loving antioxidants like vitamin E and lutein are:

Spinach

Kale

Swiss chard

By incorporating these antioxidant powerhouses into your smoothies, you can nourish your skin from within, promoting a youthful and radiant complexion.

Chapter 1: Why Everyday Smoothies?

5.2 Detoxification: A Natural Path to Healthy Skin

Detoxification is an essential process it:

Assists in the removal of toxins from your body
Enhances the immune system's capabilities
Plays a vital role in ensuring the well-being of your skin

Certain ingredients commonly found in smoothies can support your body's natural detoxification pathways, promoting clear and radiant skin.

Berries, such as

Blueberries
Raspberries
Blackberries

Are not only rich in antioxidants but also contain fiber that aids in eliminating waste and toxins from the body.

Some Leafy greens are known for their detoxifying properties. They help to cleanse and rejuvenate your skin, examples are:

Spinach
Parsley
Kale

Adding ingredients like ginger or turmeric can further enhance the detoxification process, supporting healthy liver function and reducing inflammation.

By incorporating these detoxifying ingredients into your everyday smoothies, you give your skin the love and care it deserves, helping it to thrive and radiate health.

Chapter 1: Why Everyday Smoothies?

5.3 Hydration for Healthy Skin

Maintaining proper hydration is essential for nurturing healthy and supple skin. Smoothies can play an exceptional role in keeping your body well-hydrated. Blending ingredients with high water content into your smoothies can contribute to your daily fluid intake. Some examples are:

Fruits
Vegetables
Milks

Additionally, you can enhance the hydration benefits of your smoothies by using hydrating bases like:

Coconut water
Herbal teas
Plain water

These liquids not only provide hydration but also add flavor and depth to your blends.

By staying hydrated through delicious smoothies, you can support your skin's moisture balance and achieve a radiant and dewy complexion.

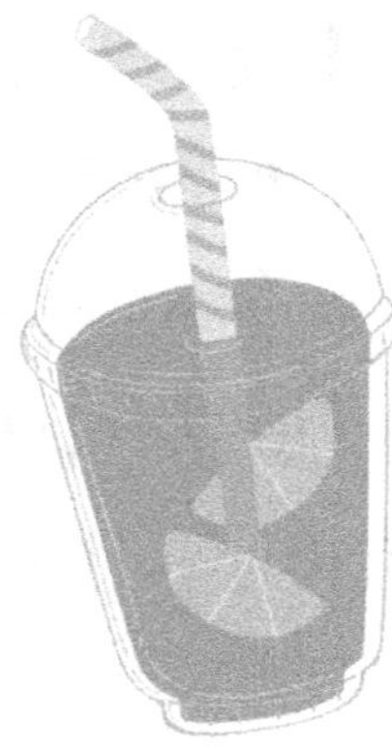

Chapter 1: Why Everyday Smoothies?

5.4 Nourish Your Skin from Within

Radiant skin starts from within, and everyday smoothies offer a powerful way to nourish your skin with the nutrients it craves. The antioxidants, detoxifying properties, and hydration benefits of smoothies work together to promote a complexion that is:

Clear

Youthful

Vibrant

To truly reap the rewards, aim to incorporate a variety of skin-loving ingredients into your smoothies. Experiment with different combinations, like:

Berry-rich blends

Green detoxifiers

Creamy Avocados

Vibrant tropical Fruits

To find the flavors and textures that please your palate and benefit your skin.

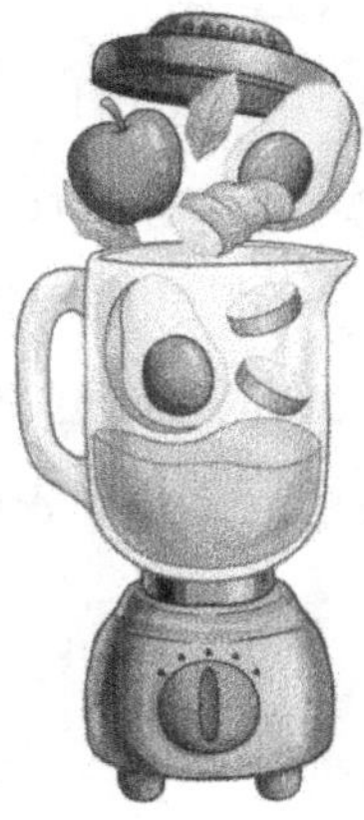

Chapter 1: Why Everyday Smoothies?

5.5 Embrace Your Natural Beauty

When you fuel your body with the wholesome goodness of everyday smoothies, you not only nourish your skin but also embrace your natural beauty. The radiant glow that comes from a well-nourished body and vibrant skin goes beyond surface-level beauty. It symbolizes your dedication to self-care and the nourishment you give from the inside out.

So, blend your way to radiant skin and natural detoxification with "Delicious Everyday Smoothies."

Unleash the power of antioxidants
Support your body's detoxification processes
Hydrate your skin from within.

Embrace your natural beauty and revel in the transformative effects that everyday smoothies can bring.

Section 5: Radiant Skin and Natural Detoxification will guide you on a journey to achieve glowing skin and support your body's detoxification processes through the magic of everyday smoothies. Be prepared to embrace your natural beauty and radiate a newfound sense of confidence.

In this chapter, we've merely skimmed the surface of the remarkable advantages that daily smoothies can bring into your life. From providing natural energy and amplifying nutrient intake to supporting digestion, weight management, and radiant skin, these blended wonders have the power to transform your well-being. So, why wait? Get a hold of your blender and prepare yourself to embark on a transformative health journey, one delightful sip at a time. Get ready to uncover the magic of everyday smoothies in the chapters that lie ahead.

Chapter 2: The Basics of Smoothie Making

Welcome to the thrilling realm of smoothie crafting! In this chapter, we'll provide you with the indispensable knowledge and tools required to concoct delectable and wholesome smoothies on every occasion. Whether you're a seasoned smoothie enthusiast or a beginner just starting your blending adventure, get ready to become a smoothie-making maestro!

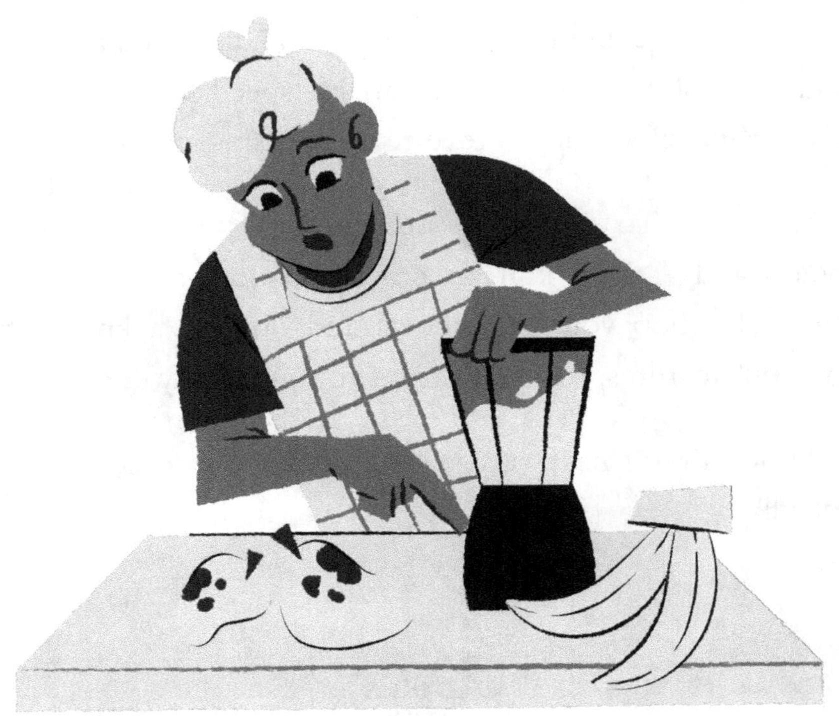

Chapter 2: The Basics of Smoothie Making

Section 1: Essential Tools and Equipment

To embark on your smoothie making journey, you'll need the right tools. We'll guide you through the essential equipment, ensuring you have everything you need to create smoothie perfection. From blenders and food processors to measuring cups and sharp knives, we'll cover all the must-haves. Discover the secrets to selecting the perfect blender for your needs and learn how to maximize its performance for silky-smooth results. Just like a chef needs the right tools in the kitchen, a smoothie enthusiast needs a few key items to create delicious and nutritious blends.

Blender: The star of the show, the blender is the cornerstone of any smoothie-making endeavor. Invest in a high-quality blender that can handle blending fruits, ice, and other ingredients smoothly. Look for features like variable speed settings and a powerful motor to ensure a consistent and silky-smooth texture in your smoothies.

Cutting Board and Knife: To effectively prepare your fruits and vegetables, having a sturdy cutting board and a sharp knife is crucial. Choose a cutting board that is large enough to comfortably chop your ingredients and opt for a knife that is suitable for cutting through various textures, from soft fruits to tough leafy greens.

Fruit Peeler: While not always necessary, a fruit peeler can come in handy for removing the skin from fruits like:

Apples

Pears

Citrus fruits

This tool helps you achieve a smoother texture in your smoothies and eliminates any unwanted bitterness or tough skin.

Chapter 2: The Basics of Smoothie Making

Section 1: Essential Tools and Equipment

Measuring Cups: Accurate measurements are key to creating well-balanced and consistent smoothies. Invest in a set of measuring cups to ensure you add the right quantities of fruits, liquids, and other ingredients to achieve the desired taste and texture.

Blender Cup or Glass: Having a designated cup or glass for your finished smoothies adds a touch of enjoyment to the experience. Choose a size that accommodates the amount of smoothie you typically make and opt for a design that brings you joy every time you take a sip.

As you progress through the Book, you'll discover the specific tools and equipment needed for each smoothie recipe. However, these five essentials are the foundation of a successful smoothie-making endeavor. Remember, having the right tools:

Makes the process more efficient

Enables you to discover boundless creative opportunities

Enhances your overall experience

Before we move on to Section 2, take a moment to gather these essential tools and equipment. They will become your trusted companions on your smoothie journey. Now that you're equipped, let's dive into the exciting world of smoothie recipes and discover the delightful flavors that await you in the pages ahead.

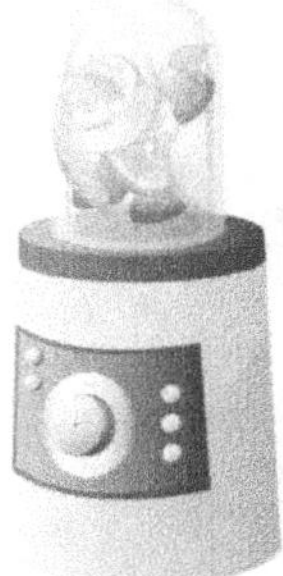

Chapter 2: The Basics of Smoothie Making

Section 2: Quality Ingredients for Flavor and Nutrition

The secret to a delightful smoothie lies in the excellence of your ingredients. We'll take a deep dive into selecting the freshest fruits, vibrant vegetables, and other nutritious add-ins that will elevate your smoothie game. Learn how to pick ripe and seasonal produce and discover the best storage methods to ensure optimum freshness and flavor. Unleash your creativity as we explore a wide range of ingredients, from sweet and tangy fruits to leafy greens, protein sources, and superfood boosters. Now is the moment to fill your pantry with a variety of nutritious ingredients, elevating your smoothies to new heights!

The world of quality ingredients helps to form the backbone of delicious and nutritious smoothies. To create truly satisfying and nourishing blends, it's important to select fresh and flavorful ingredients that provide both taste and health benefits.

Fresh Fruits and Vegetables: The cornerstone of every exceptional smoothie resides in the caliber of its fruits and vegetables. opt for ripe, seasonal produce whenever possible, as they offer peak flavor and optimal nutrient content. opt for a diverse selection of fruits and vegetables to infuse your smoothies with depth and variety. From sweet strawberries and tangy citrus fruits to nutrient-packed leafy greens like spinach, the options are endless.

Organic and Locally Sourced: Consider selecting organic fruits and vegetables to minimize exposure to pesticides and support sustainable farming practices. Additionally, sourcing ingredients locally can enhance freshness and promote the community. Check out farmers' markets or local farms to discover a range of seasonal produce for your smoothies.

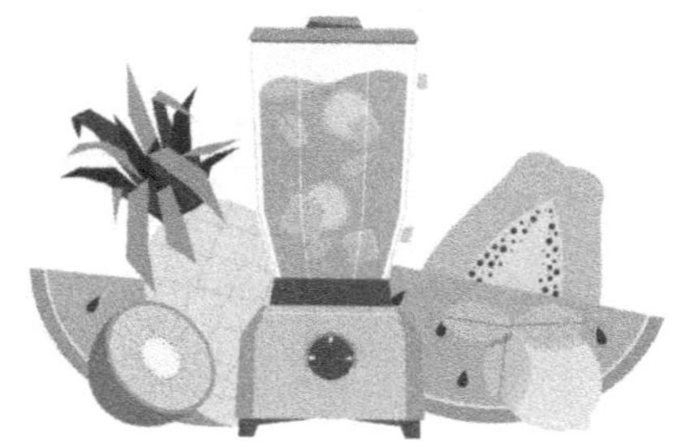

Chapter 2: The Basics of Smoothie Making

Section 2: Quality Ingredients for Flavor and Nutrition

Frozen Fruits and Vegetables. Don't underestimate the power of frozen produce. Frozen fruits and vegetables are harvested at their peak ripeness and quickly frozen, preserving their nutritional value and flavor.

They offer convenience
Extended shelf life
Serves as a budget-friendly substitute for fresh produce
Enable out-of-season fruits to be available year-round

Liquid Base: Choose a liquid base that complements the flavors of your smoothies. Unsweetened almond milk, coconut water, or plain yogurt are popular options that add creaminess and depth to your blends. Experiment with different bases to find the ones that suit your taste preferences and dietary needs.

Superfood Boosters: Elevate the nutritional profile of your smoothies by incorporating superfood boosters like:

Chia seeds
Flaxseeds
Hemp hearts
Spirulina
Matcha powder

Here are some prime illustrations of nutrient-rich additions that can amplify the health advantages of your smoothie.

Chapter 2: The Basics of Smoothie Making

Section 2: Quality Ingredients for Flavor and Nutrition

These ingredients offer an additional boost of:

Vitamins
Minerals
Antioxidants
Omega-3 fatty acids

Remember, the quality of your ingredients directly impacts your smoothies':

Taste
Texture
Nutritional value

By selecting fresh, organic, and locally sourced produce, along with incorporating superfood boosters, you'll create smoothies that not only tantalize your taste buds but also nourish your body.

In Section 3, we will put our knowledge of tools and ingredients into action as we explore a collection of mouthwatering smoothie recipes. Prepare to set your creativity free and embark on a journey of endless possibilities waiting to be explored. So, grab your blender and let's dive into the world of flavors and wellness!

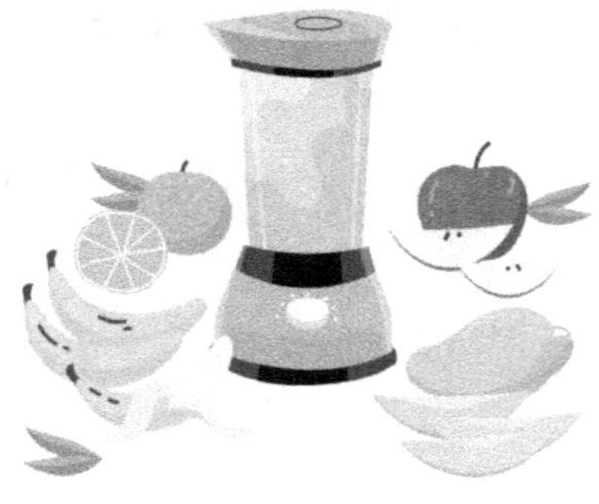

Chapter 2: The Basics of Smoothie Making

Section 3: Liquid Bases for Creaminess and Flavor

The liquid base is the foundation of a great smoothie, providing creaminess and enhancing the overall taste.

In this section, we'll explore a variety of liquid options like:

Almond milk

Coconut water

Yogurt

Herbal teas

Freshly squeezed juices

Discover the unique flavor profiles and nutritional benefits each base brings to your smoothies. We'll guide you in choosing the perfect liquid to complement your ingredients and achieve the desired texture and taste. Choosing the right liquid base is key to achieving the desired consistency and enhancing the overall taste of your blends.

Almond Milk: Almond milk is a popular choice for smoothie enthusiasts. It:

Provides Subtle nutty flavor

Provides Creamy texture

Effortlessly pairs with various fruits and vegetables

opt for unsweetened almond milk to avoid unnecessary added sugars and customize the sweetness of your smoothies according to your taste.

Chapter 2: The Basics of Smoothie Making

Section 3: Liquid Bases for Creaminess and Flavor

Coconut Water: For a tropical twist and added hydration, consider using coconut water as the base for your smoothies. Coconut water brings a:

Refreshing
Smooth texture
Slightly sweet flavor

Making it a perfect match for fruits like pineapple, mango, or berries. It's also rich in electrolytes, making it an excellent choice for:

Post-workout smoothie
Endurance smoothie
Post-illness Recovery Smoothie

Greek Yogurt: If you enjoy a thicker and more indulgent smoothie, Greek yogurt is an ideal liquid base. It adds creaminess, protein, and a tangy flavor to your blends. Greek yogurt pairs well with both sweet and tart fruits, providing a velvety texture and a boost of probiotics for gut health.

Oat Milk: Oat milk has gained popularity for its smooth and slightly sweet taste. It offers a creamy consistency that works wonderfully in smoothies, especially when combined with fruits like bananas or berries. Oat milk is also a superb option for individuals:

Who have dairy allergies or are lactose intolerant
Who are vegans or are vegetarians
Who have nut allergies

Chapter 2: The Basics of Smoothie Making

Section 3: Liquid Bases for Creaminess and Flavor

Green Tea: For an antioxidant-rich liquid base, consider incorporating brewed green tea into your smoothies. Green tea adds a subtle earthy flavor and a gentle energy boost. It pairs beautifully with fruits like citrus, pineapple, or kiwi, offering a vibrant and invigorating blend.

Fruit Juices: Freshly squeezed or cold-pressed fruit juices, such as:

Orange juice

Apple juice

Pomegranate juice

Can be used as a flavorful liquid base. They add natural sweetness and enhance the fruity taste of your smoothies. opt for unsweetened options and be mindful of the sugar content in fruit juices.

Remember, the choice of your liquid base can significantly influence the texture, taste, and nutritional profile of your smoothies. Experiment with different options to find the ones that complement your preferred fruits, vegetables, and superfood boosters.

In Section 4, we will bring together the essential tools, quality ingredients, and liquid bases to create a variety of tantalizing smoothie recipes. Get ready to blend, sip, and savor the deliciousness that awaits you. Let's continue our smoothie adventure and explore the art of flavor combinations!

Chapter 2: The Basics of Smoothie Making

Section 4: Sweeteners and Flavor Enhancers

While fruits naturally bring sweetness to your smoothies, you might occasionally want to add an extra touch of flavor or sweetness. We'll delve into the world of natural sweeteners and flavor enhancers, exploring options like:

Honey

Maple syrup

Dates

Spices

Master the art of achieving the ideal harmony between sweetness and various flavor elements and explore techniques for tailoring your smoothies to perfectly match your unique taste preferences. It's time to infuse your creations with irresistible flavors that will leave you craving more.

Natural Sweeteners

Honey: A classic natural sweetener, honey adds a rich, sweet taste to your smoothies. Choose raw, unprocessed honey for maximum health benefits.

Maple Syrup: With its distinctive caramel flavor, maple syrup is a popular sweetener for smoothies. opt for pure, organic maple syrup to experience its full depth of flavor.

Medjool Dates: Dates are a delicious and nutritious way to sweeten your smoothies naturally. They provide a pleasant caramel-like taste and a creamy texture when blended.

Chapter 2: The Basics of Smoothie Making

Section 4: Sweeteners and Flavor Enhancers

Spices and Extracts:

Cinnamon: A versatile spice that adds warmth and depth to your smoothies. Just a sprinkle of cinnamon can transform your blend into a comforting treat reminiscent of freshly baked goods.

Vanilla Extract: Enhance your smoothies with a delightful aroma and subtle sweetness by adding a few drops of pure vanilla extract. opt for high-quality, genuine vanilla extract to achieve the finest outcomes.

Almond Extract: Elevate your smoothies with a nutty and aromatic twist by incorporating a hint of almond extract. It pairs exceptionally well with fruits like cherries, peaches, or berries.

Citrus Zest and Juices:

Lemon Zest: Grate some fresh lemon zest into your smoothies to add a bright, tangy flavor. The zest provides a burst of citrusy freshness that complements a wide range of fruits

Lime Juice: Squeeze a splash of lime juice into your smoothies for a zesty and refreshing kick. Lime pairs beautifully with tropical fruits like mango, pineapple, or kiwi.

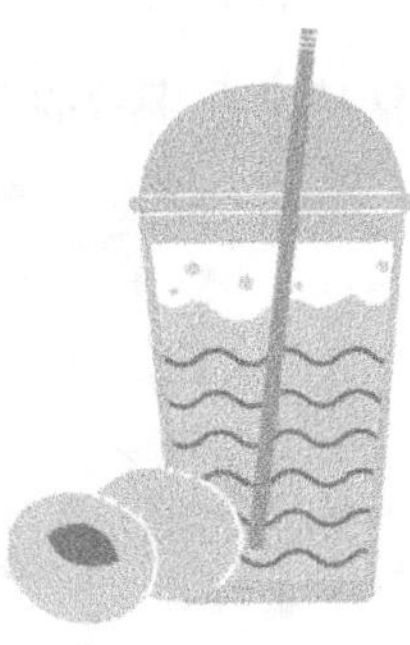

Chapter 2: The Basics of Smoothie Making

Section 4: Sweeteners and Flavor Enhancers

Nut Butters:

Peanut Butter: Smooth and luxurious, this delightful spread infuses your smoothies with a rich, nutty taste and a velvety consistency. Choose natural peanut butter without added sugars or oils for a healthier option.

Almond Butter: opt for a gentle and subtly sweet flavor by choosing almond butter. Its seamless blending with fruits and vegetables delivers a smooth and creamy texture to your creations.

Keep in mind that moderation is key when using sweeteners and flavor enhancers to ensure your smoothie remains:

Balanced
Nutritious
Enjoyable

Tailor the quantities to your taste preferences and don't hesitate to experiment with various options, allowing you to craft distinct and delightful flavor combinations.

In Section 5, we will put our knowledge of essential tools, quality ingredients, liquid bases, and sweeteners to work as we dive into a collection of delectable smoothie recipes. Get ready to blend, savor, and enjoy the symphony of flavors that await you. Let's continue our smoothie adventure and unleash your creativity in the kitchen!

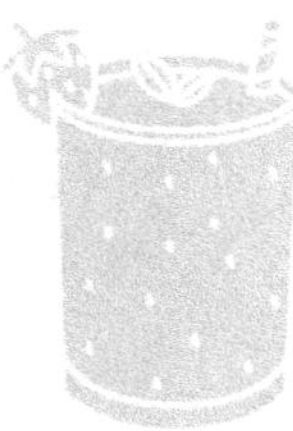

Chapter 2: The Basics of Smoothie Making

Section 5: Blending Techniques and Tips

Blending is an art form, and in this section, we'll share expert tips and techniques to achieve the perfect smoothie consistency. From layering your ingredients strategically to achieve even blending to adjusting the blending time for different ingredients, we'll equip you with the knowledge to master the art of smoothie blending. Say goodbye to lumps, chunks, and uneven textures as you create velvety-smooth, drinkable masterpieces every time

.Mastering the blending process is key to creating smoothie mixes that showcase the full potential of your ingredients and are:

Smooth

Creamy

Well-incorporated

Layering Ingredients:

Start by adding the liquid base to your blender, followed by the leafy greens (if using any) and then the fruits, superfood boosters, sweeteners, and flavor enhancers. Layering the ingredients in this order helps ensure proper blending and prevents ingredients from getting stuck at the bottom of the blender.

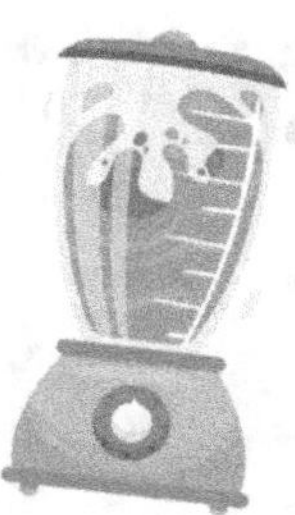

Chapter 2: The Basics of Smoothie Making

Section 5: Blending Techniques and Tips

Blending Time and Speed:

Blend your smoothie on high speed for approximately 30 to 60 seconds or until all the ingredients are well combined and you achieve a smooth, uniform texture. Steer clear of over-blending, as it can result in:

Excessive heat

Oxidation

Diluted texture

Which may affect the taste and nutritional value of your smoothie.

Adding Ice:

If you prefer a chilled and refreshing smoothie, consider adding a handful of ice cubes to the blender. This helps to cool down the temperature and gives your smoothie a satisfying frosty texture. However, if using frozen fruits, you may not need to add additional ice.

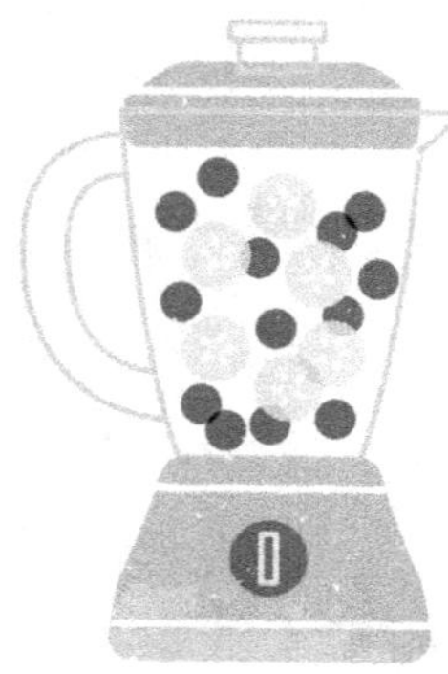

Chapter 2: The Basics of Smoothie Making

Section 5: Blending Techniques and Tips

Adjusting Consistency:

If your smoothie turns out too thick, gradually add small amounts of liquid such as:

Water

Juice

Almond milk

Until you achieve your desired consistency.

On the other hand, if your smoothie is too thin, add more of the following to thicken it up:

Fruits or vegetables

Chia seeds or flaxseeds

Yogurt or nut butter

Customizing Texture:

Tailor the texture of your smoothie to your preference. If you enjoy a silky-smooth consistency, blend for a longer duration. For a chunkier texture with small fruit pieces, blend for a shorter time or use the pulse function on your blender.

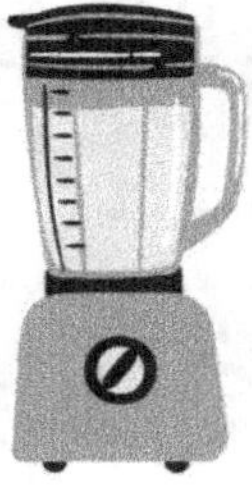

Chapter 2: The Basics of Smoothie Making

Section 5: Blending Techniques and Tips

Experimenting with Variations:

Don't be afraid to experiment with different:

Ingredients
Quantities
Techniques

Discover your own signature blends by exploring various fruits, vegetables, superfood boosters, and flavor profiles. Keep a record of your favorite creations to revisit and share with others.

Remember, blending techniques are an art form that allows you to customize your smoothies to suit your personal taste and texture preferences.

Embrace the creative process
Have lots of fun
Let your imagination run wild

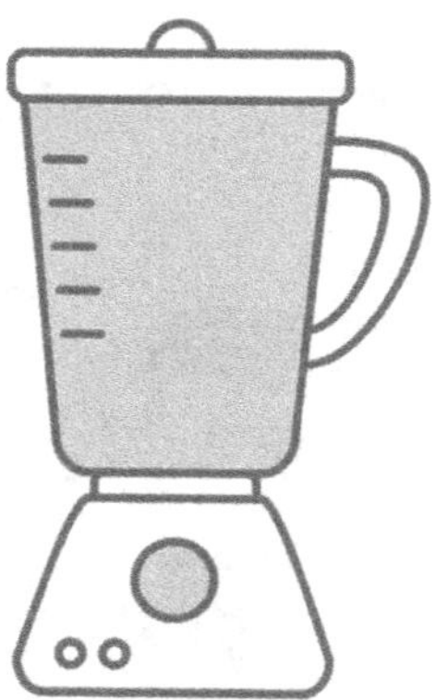

Chapter 2: The Basics of Smoothie Making

Section 5: Blending Techniques and Tips

Congratulations! You've now mastered the basics of smoothie making.

You're ready to create smoothies that will delight your taste buds and nourish your body, armed with:

**The right tools
Quality ingredients
Expert techniques**

In the upcoming chapters, we shall embark on an exciting 7-day smoothie challenge, immersing ourselves in a delightful array of flavors and discovering the remarkable impact of incorporating daily smoothies into your routine. Get set to blend your path to a healthier and more vibrant self!

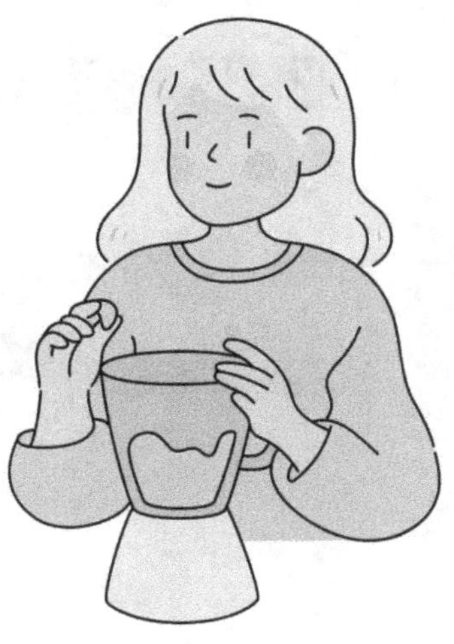

Chapter 3: The 7-Day Smoothie Challenge

Welcome to the heart of our Book, we will now embark on a 7-day journey to explore the tantalizing world of everyday smoothies. Together we will explore a new flavor adventure each day, this will allow you to indulge in a variety of delectable smoothie combinations. Get ready to awaken your taste buds and nourish your body with the power of these delightful creations.

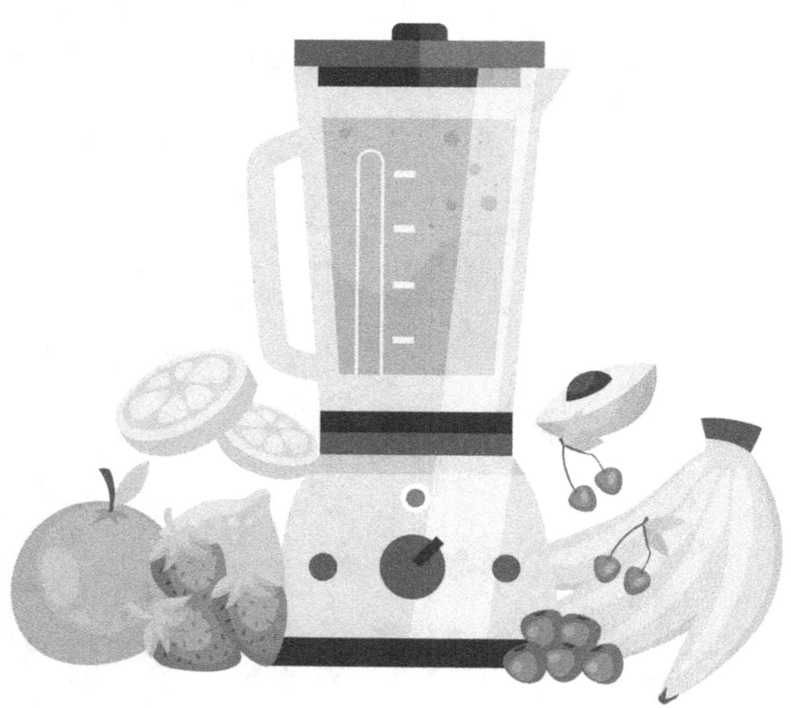

Chapter 3: The 7-Day Smoothie Challenge

Day 1: Apple Banana Smoothie

Our challenge begins with the classic combination of apples and bananas. Dive into the crisp sweetness of apples and the creamy texture of bananas as they blend harmoniously to create a smoothie that will leave you craving more. We'll provide you with a simple recipe to start your journey and offer variations to suit different flavor profiles and dietary preferences. Get ready to kickstart your mornings with this invigorating blend!

For our 7-day smoothie challenge we focus on creating healthy and delicious smoothies steering clear of processed sugar.

Instead, we rely on the natural sweetness of various fruits like:

Dates

Red grapes

Pineapples

Apples

Bananas

With these sweet treasures we have the perfect foundation for our smoothies, allowing us to create flavorful concoctions without compromising our commitment to a healthy lifestyle.

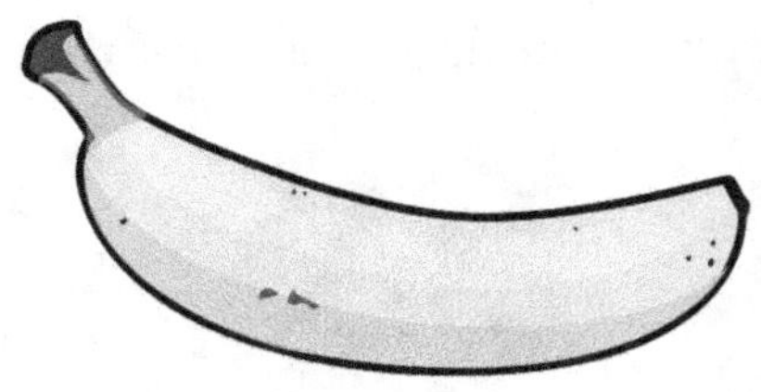

Chapter 3: The 7-Day Smoothie Challenge

Day 1: Apple Banana Smoothie

We also explore natural flavoring alternatives to elevate our smoothies to new heights. Think:

**Vanilla
Almond extract
Cocoa powder**

And aromatic spices like:

**Clove
Cinnamon
Nutmeg**

With these additions we can add a burst of complexity to the Apple Banana Smoothie, transforming it into a truly extraordinary treat.

Our initial focus maybe currently on fruit smoothies, but we promise you that there is much more to come. Our taste buds crave the bitter, the sour, and the tangy, and we will surely explore those flavors in our 7-day challenge. Additionally, our green side is beckoning, and we can't wait to unveil our recipe for vibrant green smoothies. Stay tuned for more exciting blends coming your way soon!

But for now, let's dive into the delightful world of the Apple Banana Smoothie. These two fruits create an impeccable synergy, resulting in a smoothie that is bursting with irresistible flavor.

Chapter 3: The 7-Day Smoothie Challenge

Day 1: Apple Banana Smoothie:
The Perfect Fusion of Sweetness and Creaminess

Welcome to Day 1 of our seven-day smoothie challenge! Today, we kick off our journey with a delightful blend of two beloved fruits – apples and bananas. The combination of these:

Sweet

Creamy

Wholesome

Fruits will create a delicious smoothie packed with essential nutrients to start your day off right. Let's dive into the recipe!

Ingredients:

1-2 apples (any variety you prefer)

1 ripe banana

1 cup of almond milk. (Unsweetened)

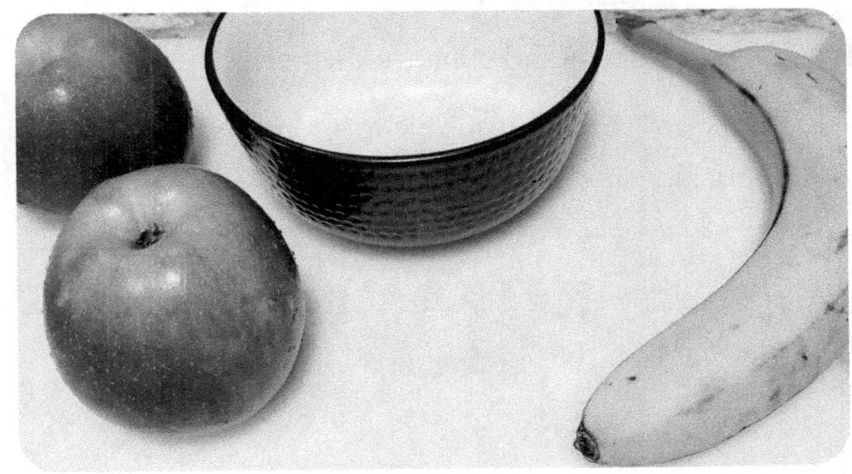

Chapter 3: The 7-Day Smoothie Challenge

Day 1: Apple Banana Smoothie:
The Perfect Fusion of Sweetness and Creaminess

Instructions:

Start by preparing your ingredients. Core and chop the apple into small pieces, and peel the ripe banana.

Place the unsweetened almond milk into the blender.

Place the chopped apple and banana into your blender.

Blend all the ingredients together. Blend at high speed until you reach a smooth and creamy texture.

Give the smoothie a taste and adjust the sweetness or thickness by adding more apple or almond milk if desired.

Pour the smoothie into a glass or jar, and feel free to garnish with:

A Sprinkle of cinnamon

A slice of apple

A dusting of nutmeg

To add an additional burst of flavor and enhance the overall presentation.

Take a moment to appreciate the beautiful blend of colors and aromas before enjoying your refreshing and nourishing apple banana smoothie.

Chapter 3: The 7-Day Smoothie Challenge

Day 1: Apple Banana Smoothie:
The Perfect Fusion of Sweetness and Creaminess

This delightful concoction combines the natural sweetness of apples with the creamy texture of bananas, resulting in a smoothie that is:

Perfectly balanced
Satisfying
Irresistible

The apple adds a touch of tartness and a subtle crunch, while the banana lends its creamy goodness and an abundance of potassium and fiber.

Sip on this delicious creation as:

A quick and nourishing breakfast
A satisfying snack
A post-workout refuel

The combination of:

Vitamins
Minerals
Antioxidants

In this apple banana smoothie will provide you with a boost of energy and support your overall well-being.

Chapter 3: The 7-Day Smoothie Challenge

Day 1: Apple Banana Smoothie:
The Perfect Fusion of Sweetness and Creaminess

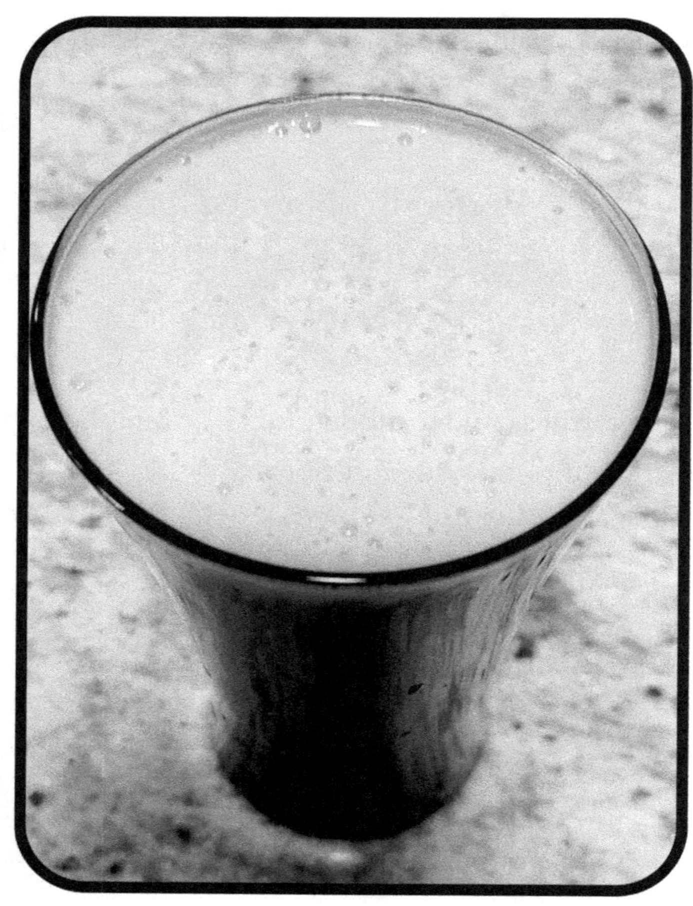

Stay tuned for Day 2 of our seven-day smoothie challenge, where we'll introduce another tantalizing recipe to keep you on track toward a healthier and more vibrant lifestyle. Don't forget to share your smoothie creations and experiences with our thriving community at www.modernlivingguide.com. Let's inspire and support each other on this wonderful journey of continuous improvement!

Feel free to use the journal section provided in the resource section at the back of the book to jot down your notes and experiences as you continue to read.

Chapter 3: The 7-Day Smoothie Challenge

Day 2: Apple Smoothie

Let's continue our exploration of apples. We will keep on with discovering the versatility of apple-based smoothies as we showcase a range of creative flavor combinations. From refreshing green apple and cucumber to indulgent apple cinnamon, you'll be amazed at the endless possibilities. Let fly your imagination and create a signature apple smoothie that reflects your unique taste.

Welcome back to our fruity smoothie 7-day challenge! We're diving deeper into the world of fruit smoothies, exploring new ways to add healthy sweetness without relying on processed or refined sugars. Allow us to introduce you to some alternative sweeteners that will elevate your smoothie game. Imagine infusing your blends with the rich flavors of:

Vanilla

Almond extract

Cocoa powder

Or aromatic spices like clove. And let's not forget one of our personal favorites: cinnamon spice. Adding a pinch of cinnamon to your smoothie will transport you to a realm of:

Cozy comfort

Aromatic delight

Nostalgic bliss

Reminiscent of enjoying a slice of warm apple pie.

Chapter 3: The 7-Day Smoothie Challenge

Day 2: Apple Smoothie

Cinnamon spice isn't just about adding incredible flavor; it also offers numerous health benefits. Packed with properties like:

Antioxidants
Anti-inflammatory
Anti-diabetic

Cinnamon brings an extra layer of goodness to your already healthy smoothie. The addition of cinnamon spice takes your apple smoothie to new heights of flavor and nourishment. By combining:

The natural sweetness of apples
The warm embrace of cinnamon spice
The creaminess of almond milk

This smoothie captures the comforting essence of a freshly baked apple pie made at home. Perhaps you might even call it an apple pie smoothie we'll leave that decision up to you.

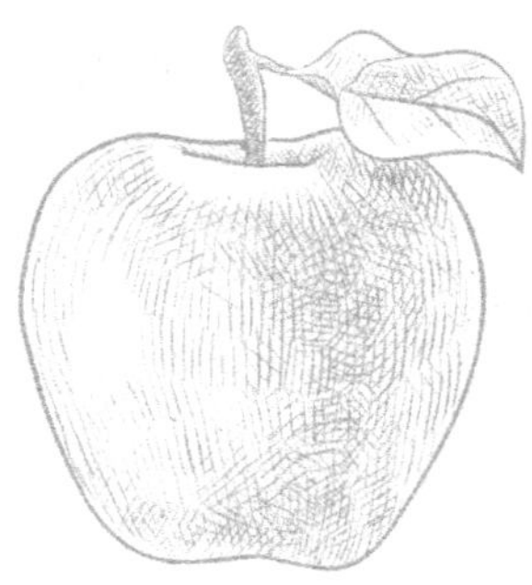

Chapter 3: The 7-Day Smoothie Challenge

Day 2: Apple Smoothie:
Indulge in the Homey Delight of Apple Pie

You've reached Day 2 of our seven-day smoothie challenge! We are going to shine the spotlight on the versatile apple today. Apples are not just tasty; they are also loaded with:

Essential nutrients
Fiber
Natural goodness

Making them an excellent addition to any smoothie. Get ready to indulge in the refreshing flavors of our apple smoothie!

Ingredients:

2 apples (any variety you prefer)

1 cup of almond milk. (unsweetened)

A sprinkle of ground cinnamon (optional)

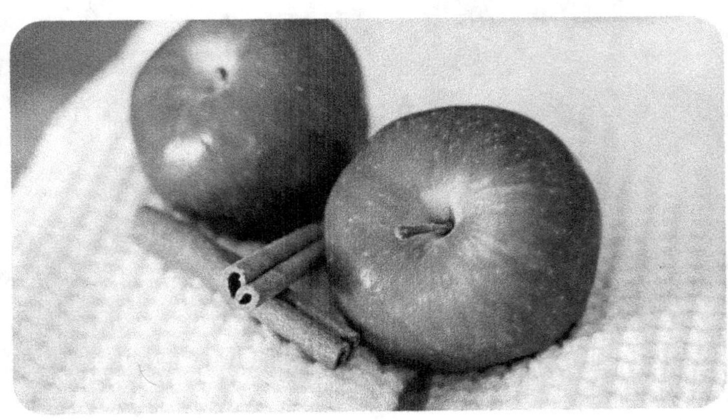

Chapter 3: The 7-Day Smoothie Challenge

Day 2: Apple Smoothie:
Indulge in the Homey Delight of Apple Pie

Instructions:

Begin by preparing the apples. Core and chop them into smaller pieces, leaving the skin on for added fiber and nutrients.

Place the unsweetened almond milk into the blender.

Place the chopped apples into your blender.

For an extra touch of:

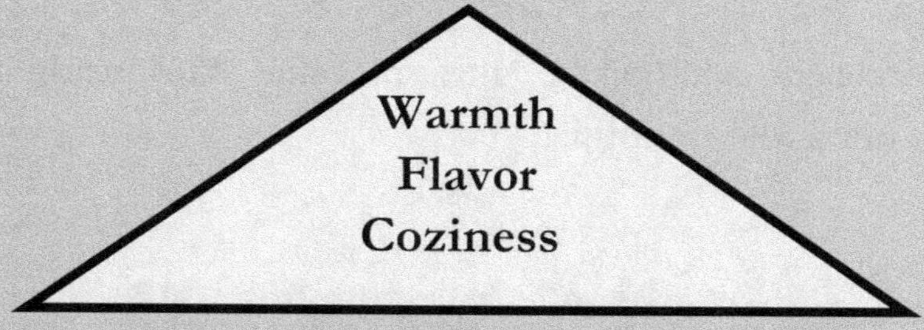

Add a sprinkle of ground cinnamon.

Blend all the ingredients together. Blend at high speed until you reach a smooth and creamy texture.

Give the smoothie a taste and adjust the sweetness or thickness by adding more apple or almond milk if desired.

Pour the smoothie into a glass or jar, and feel free to garnish with:

Chapter 3: The 7-Day Smoothie Challenge

Day 2: Apple Smoothie:
Indulge in the Homey Delight of Apple Pie

Take a moment to admire the beautiful blend of colors and aromas before savoring your revitalizing apple smoothie.

This apple smoothie captures the homely feeling of indulging in a slice of apple pie and is a celebration of the fruit's:

Natural sweetness

Crisp texture

Comforting aroma

The combination of apples and almond milk creates a creamy base, while the hint of cinnamon adds:

Delightful warmth

Complexity

Richness

To the flavor profile. As you take each sip, feel the invigorating burst of apple goodness awaken your senses and nourish your body.

Enjoy this refreshing apple smoothie as a:

Guilt-free dessert

Mid-day pick-me-up

Delicious breakfast option

Chapter 3: The 7-Day Smoothie Challenge

Day 2: Apple Smoothie:
Indulge in the Homey Delight of Apple Pie

Apples are not only hydrating but also rich in:

Antioxidants
Vitamins
Dietary fiber

Providing you with:

A boost of energy
Vitality
A sense of rejuvenation

Supporting your overall well-being.

We hope you relish the:

Simplicity
Wholesomeness
Delightful flavors

Of this apple smoothie.

Chapter 3: The 7-Day Smoothie Challenge

Day 2: Apple Smoothie:
Indulge in the Homey Delight of Apple Pie

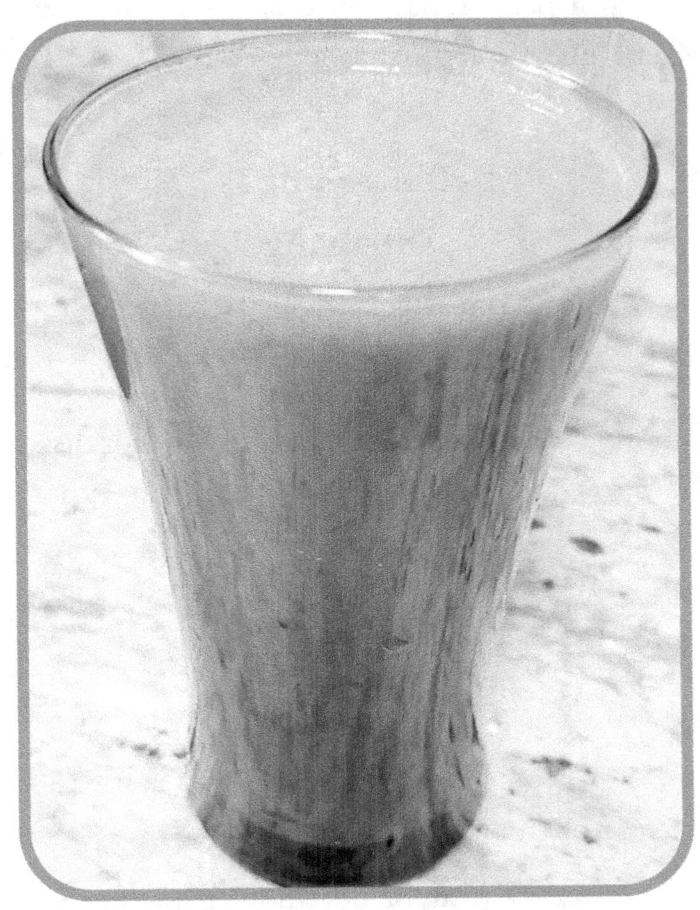

Keep going for Day 3 of our seven-day smoothie challenge, where we will introduce another tantalizing recipe to keep your taste buds intrigued and your health journey on track.

Don't forget to share your smoothie experiences and join our thriving community at www.modernlivingguide.com. Let's inspire and uplift one another on this incredible path to continuous improvement!

Chapter 3: The 7-Day Smoothie Challenge

Day 3: Banana Pear Smoothie

We venture into the world of pears today. We'll be combining pears' delicate flavor with the creaminess of bananas. The result? A smoothie that is:

Refreshing

Satisfying

Absolutely delightful

During the 7-day smoothie challenge, take a moment to discover and explore the nutritional benefits of pears and bananas. Also, you can experiment with additional ingredients like:

Ginger

Cinnamon

Nutmeg

To add depth and complexity to your blend. Indulge in the velvety goodness of this delightful combination.

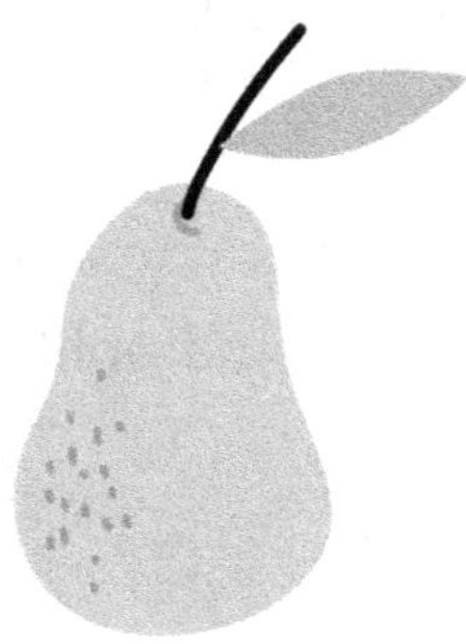

Chapter 3: The 7-Day Smoothie Challenge

Day 3: Banana Pear Smoothie

Welcome back to our journey through the world of smoothies that are:

Sweet

Nutritious

Wholesome

We're diving into the delightful combination of bananas and pears. Get ready to experience a level of creamy sweetness that will transport you to smoothie heaven.

Pear is a fruit beloved worldwide, known for its:

Diverse colors

Shapes

Rich nutrients

It boasts a natural sweetness, although you can find less sweet varieties if you prefer. On the other hand, ripe bananas offer:

Sweetness

Creaminess

Exceptional nutritional value

We're taking our passion for fruit smoothies to new heights with the banana pear smoothie. This delightful blend captures the perfect balance between:

Creamy texture

Indulgent richness

Luscious sweetness

Bringing back memories of a traditional vanilla milkshake. This recipe allows us to satisfy our sweet side while maintaining a healthy approach. We are happy to share.

Chapter 3: The 7-Day Smoothie Challenge

Day 3: Banana Pear Smoothie: Indulge in Creamy Sweetness

Welcome to Day 3 of our seven-day smoothie challenge! We invite you to indulge in the delightful combination of bananas and pears smoothie today that is refreshing and creamy. You can create a harmonious blend that will leave your taste buds craving for more by combining:

The natural sweetness of the bananas

The subtle flavor of pears

The silkiness of your liquid base

Let's dive into the recipe!

Ingredients:

1 ripe banana

1 ripe pear

1 cup of almond milk. (unsweetened)

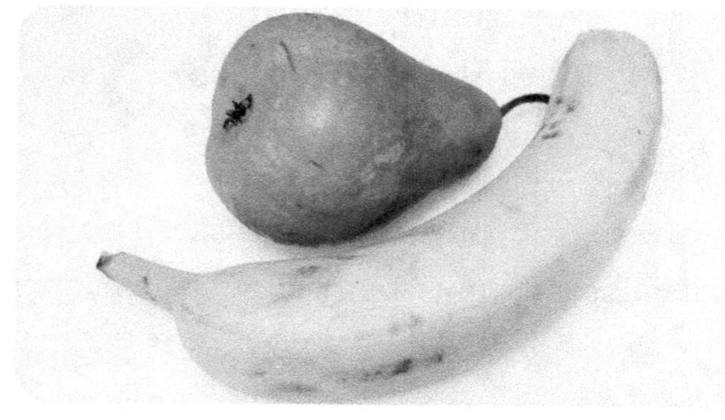

Chapter 3: The 7-Day Smoothie Challenge

Day 3: Banana Pear Smoothie: Indulge in Creamy Sweetness

Instructions:

Begin by peeling the ripe banana and pear, removing any seeds or stems.

Chop the banana and pear into smaller pieces.

Place the unsweetened almond milk into the blender.

Place the chopped banana and pear into your blender.

Blend all the ingredients together. Blend at high speed until you reach a smooth and creamy texture.

Give the smoothie a taste and adjust the sweetness or thickness by adding more banana or almond milk if desired.

Pour the banana pear smoothie into a glass or jar, and consider garnishing with a slice of fresh pear for an elegant touch.

Take a moment to appreciate the beautiful blend of flavors and textures before enjoying your revitalizing banana pear smoothie.

Chapter 3: The 7-Day Smoothie Challenge

Day 3: Banana Pear Smoothie: Indulge in Creamy Sweetness

This smoothie is a celebration of the delicate flavors and natural sweetness of both bananas and pears. The creaminess of the bananas pairs perfectly with the juicy and slightly grainy texture of the pears, creating a beverage that is:

Satisfying
Wholesome
Nourishing

Savor each sip of this banana pear smoothie as it provides you with essential nutrients such as:

Potassium
Fiber
Vitamin C

Whether you enjoy it as a:

Quick breakfast on the go
Mid-day snack
Post-workout replenishment

This smoothie is sure to keep you feeling:

Energized
Revitalized
Satisfied

Chapter 3: The 7-Day Smoothie Challenge

Day 3: Banana Pear Smoothie: Indulge in Creamy Sweetness

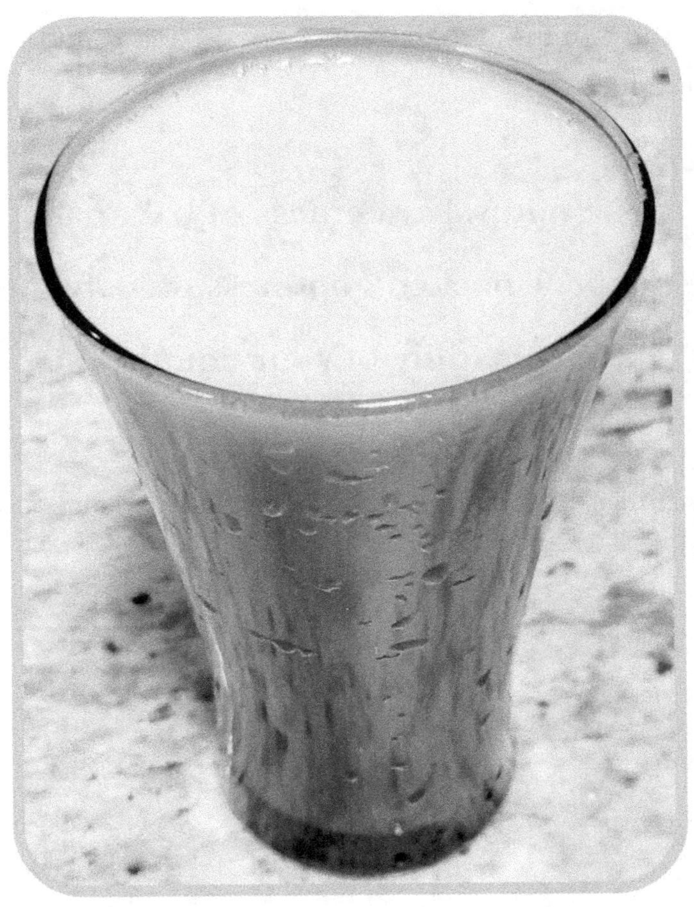

Stay tuned for Day 4 of our seven-day smoothie challenge, where we'll introduce another tantalizing recipe to keep your taste buds intrigued and your health journey on track. Don't forget to share your smoothie experiences and join our thriving community at www.modernlivingguide.com. Let's continue to inspire and support one another on this incredible path to continuous improvement!

Chapter 3: The 7-Day Smoothie Challenge

Day 4: Banana Smoothie with Spinach

Get ready to embrace the vibrant green goodness of a banana and spinach smoothie. This powerhouse blend combines:

The natural sweetness of bananas

The nutrient-packed goodness of leafy greens

The versatility of your liquid base

We'll share tips for seamlessly incorporating spinach into your smoothies, ensuring that each sip is packed with:

Vitamins

Minerals

Antioxidants

This could become your new favorite go to recipe, don't be surprised!

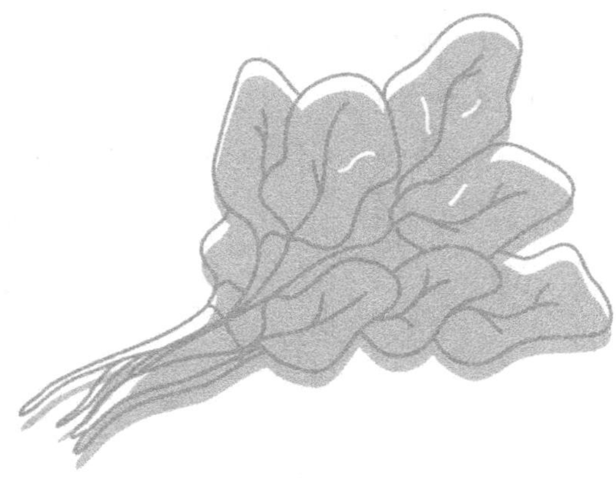

Chapter 3: The 7-Day Smoothie Challenge

Day 4: Banana Smoothie with Spinach

Welcome to the world of smoothie exploration! Are you in the mood for:

A fruit smoothie

A green smoothie

A delightful blend of both

Discover the flavors that will satisfy your taste buds dive in now.

From classic banana smoothies to refreshing strawberry blends, there's a fruity concoction to suit every palate. And why not combine both into a delightful strawberry banana smoothie? The choice is yours, we're excited to be a guide.

On the other hand, if you're seeking the vibrant green goodness of a green smoothie look no further. We've curated a green smoothie recipe, designed to:

Invigorate your senses

Boost your energy

Nourish your body

We're thrilled to share an easy-to-make, delicious smoothie featuring a superstar ingredient: spinach. But don't worry this isn't your ordinary spinach smoothie. We've infused it with the flavors of our beloved banana smoothie to create a fusion of fruity delight and wholesome greens.

Chapter 3: The 7-Day Smoothie Challenge

Day 4: Banana Smoothie with Spinach:
The Perfect Fusion of Greens and Fruity Delight

Welcome to Day 4 of our seven-day smoothie challenge! Today, we're going to take your smoothie game to the next level by introducing a combination that is:

Vibrant

Refreshing

Nutritious

The Banana Smoothie with Spinach. This invigorating blend of creamy bananas and nutrient-packed spinach will provide you with:

Burst of energy

Vitality

Nourishment

Let's dive into the recipe!

Ingredients:

1 ripe banana

1 cup of fresh spinach leaves

1 cup of almond milk. (unsweetened)

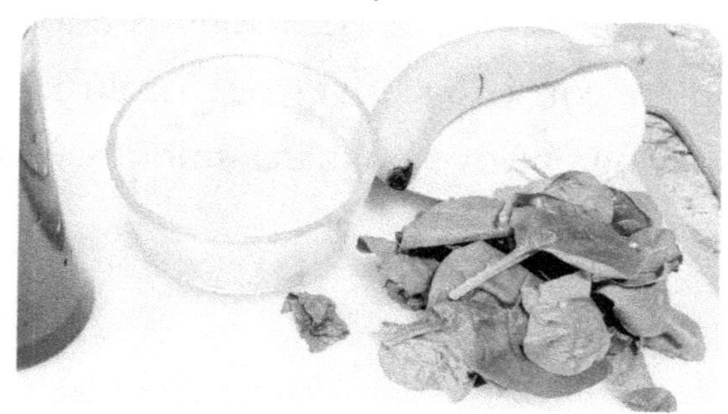

Chapter 3: The 7-Day Smoothie Challenge

Day 4: Banana Smoothie with Spinach:
The Perfect Fusion of Greens and Fruity Delight

Instructions.

Begin by peeling the ripe banana. Cut it into smaller pieces.

Wash the fresh spinach leaves thoroughly and remove any tough stems.

Place the unsweetened almond milk into the blender.

Place the banana and spinach leaves into your blender.

Blend all the ingredients together. Blend on high speed until you achieve a smooth and vibrant green mixture.

Give the smoothie a taste and adjust the sweetness or thickness by adding more banana or almond milk if desired.

Pour the banana smoothie with spinach into a glass or jar, and take a moment to marvel at the beautiful green hue before sipping your revitalizing creation.

Chapter 3: The 7-Day Smoothie Challenge

Day 4: Banana Smoothie with Spinach:
The Perfect Fusion of Greens and Fruity Delight

This smoothie is the perfect fusion of creamy sweetness from the bananas and the nutritional powerhouse of fresh spinach. The mild taste of the spinach is beautifully balanced by the natural sweetness of the bananas, creating a harmonious blend that is:

Delicious

Invigorating

Nourishing

As you enjoy this vibrant smoothie, you're not only treating yourself to a delightful beverage, but you're also fueling your body with:

Essential vitamins

Minerals

Antioxidants

The spinach provides an excellent source of:

Iron

Calcium

Vitamins A and C

while the bananas offer:

Potassium

Vitamin B6

Dietary fiber

Chapter 3: The 7-Day Smoothie Challenge

Day 4: Banana Smoothie with Spinach:
The Perfect Fusion of Greens and Fruity Delight

Whether you choose to enjoy this smoothie as:

A morning boost

A mid-day refresher

A post-workout replenishment

It will leave you feeling:

Refreshed

Revitalized

Ready to tackle the day ahead

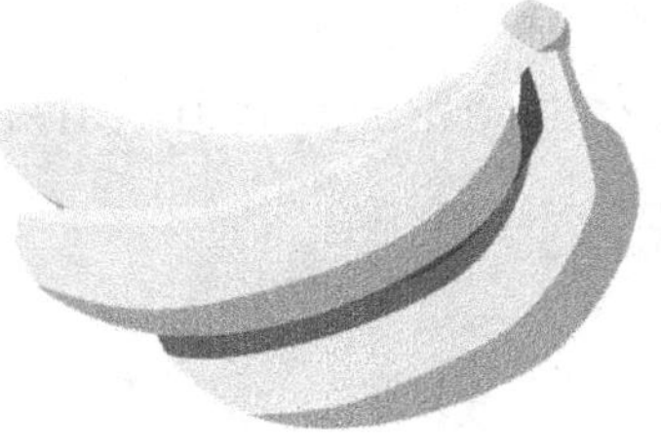

Chapter 3: The 7-Day Smoothie Challenge

Day 4: Banana Smoothie with Spinach:
The Perfect Fusion of Greens and Fruity Delight

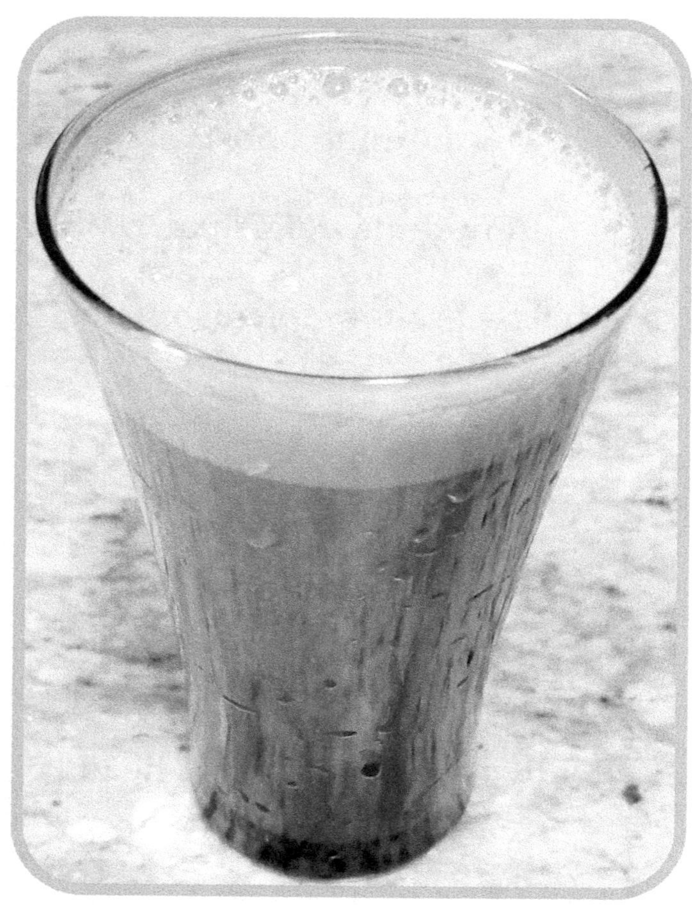

Stay tuned for Day 5 of our seven-day smoothie challenge, where we'll introduce another tantalizing recipe to keep your taste buds intrigued and your health journey on track. Don't forget to share your smoothie experiences and join our thriving community at www.modernlivingguide.com. Let's continue to inspire and support one another on this incredible path to continuous improvement!

Chapter 3: The 7-Day Smoothie Challenge

Day 5: Orange Banana Smoothie

Welcome back to our exploration of the wonderful world of smoothies! We're continuing to dive into the realm of sweetness, but not just any sweetness healthy sweetness derived from the vibrant flavors of fruits. Join us as we continue to discover the incredible taste profiles and endless possibilities of fruit smoothies.

It's time to infuse a zesty citrus twist into your smoothie repertoire. Join us as we explore the delightful combination of oranges and bananas. Revel in the tangy sweetness and experience the immune-boosting properties of this dynamic duo. We'll offer suggestions for adding a touch of warmth with ingredients like:

Turmeric
Cinnamon
Coconut flakes

Taking your orange banana smoothie to new heights of flavor and nutrition.

When it comes to crafting smoothies that are:

Sweet
Refreshing
Delicious

The abundance of fruits available to us is truly awe inspiring. Each fruit brings its own benefits like:

Unique flavor
Texture
Nutrition

Allowing us to craft a wide array of mouthwatering recipes.

Chapter 3: The 7-Day Smoothie Challenge

Day 5: Orange Banana Smoothie

Introducing: the orange banana smoothie. Bursting with refreshing citrus flavors, this smoothie belongs on the list of must-try fruit smoothies. The combination of orange and banana creates a delightful balance of:

Tanginess

Creaminess

Sweetness

Making it an incredibly delicious and refreshing treat.

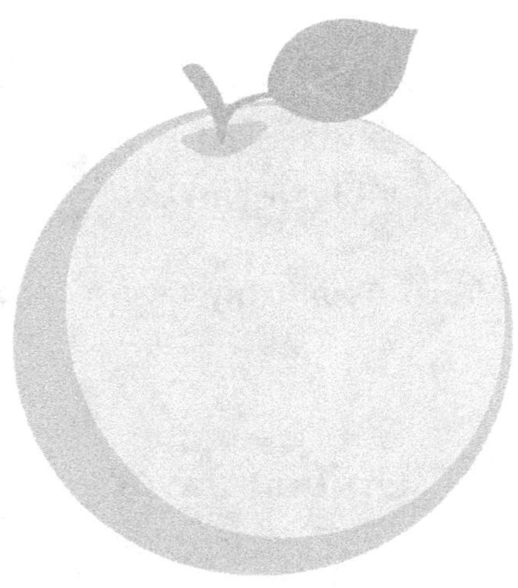

Chapter 3: The 7-Day Smoothie Challenge

Day 5: Orange Banana Smoothie:
A Burst of Refreshing Sweetness

Welcome to Day 5 of our seven-day smoothie challenge! Today, we have the Orange Banana Smoothie which is a treat that is:

Refreshing

Vivacious

Citrusy

This vibrant blend of oranges and bananas will transport you to a sunny paradise while providing a burst of vitamin C and natural sweetness. Let's dive into the recipe!

Ingredients:

3 oranges (peeled and segmented)

½ ripe banana

1 cup of almond milk. (Unsweetened)

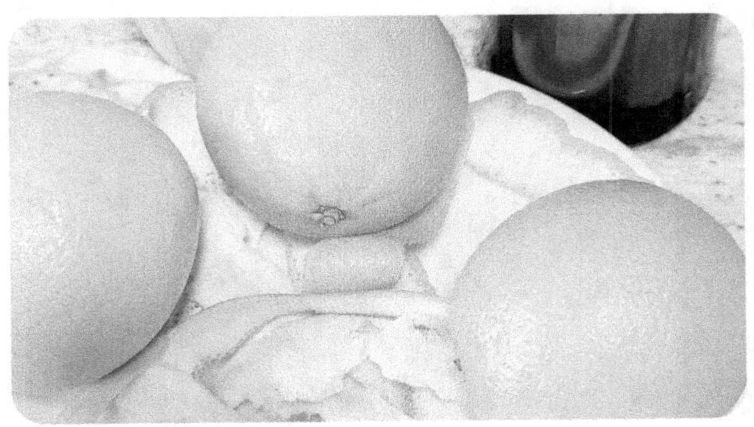

Chapter 3: The 7-Day Smoothie Challenge

Day 5: Orange Banana Smoothie:
A Burst of Refreshing Sweetness

Instructions:

Begin by peeling and segmenting the oranges, removing any seeds.

Peel the ripe banana. Cut it into smaller pieces.

Place the unsweetened almond milk into the blender.

Place the orange segments and banana into your blender.

Blend all the ingredients together. Blend at high speed until you reach a smooth and creamy texture.

Give the smoothie a taste and adjust the sweetness or thickness by adding more orange or almond milk if desired.

Pour the orange banana smoothie into a glass or jar, and take a moment to appreciate the vibrant color and invigorating aroma before sipping your citrus-infused creation.

Chapter 3: The 7-Day Smoothie Challenge

Day 5: Orange Banana Smoothie:
A Burst of Refreshing Sweetness

This smoothie is a delightful blend of:

Tangy oranges

Nutty almond milk

Creamy bananas

Creating a harmonious balance of flavors.

The oranges provide a refreshing burst of vitamin C and antioxidants

The bananas contribute a creamy texture and natural sweetness

The milk adds a nutty undertone and smooth consistency

As you savor each sip of this orange banana smoothie, you're:

Treating yourself to a tropical delight

Boosting your immune system

Supporting overall well-being

The combination of citrus and potassium-rich bananas will leave you feeling refreshed and revitalized.

Chapter 3: The 7-Day Smoothie Challenge

Day 5: Orange Banana Smoothie:
A Burst of Refreshing Sweetness

Enjoy this rejuvenating smoothie as a:

Morning pick-me-up

Revitalizing mid-day snack

Post-workout refuel

It's the perfect way to brighten your day and satisfy your taste buds with this goodness that is:

Zesty

Creamy

Invigorating

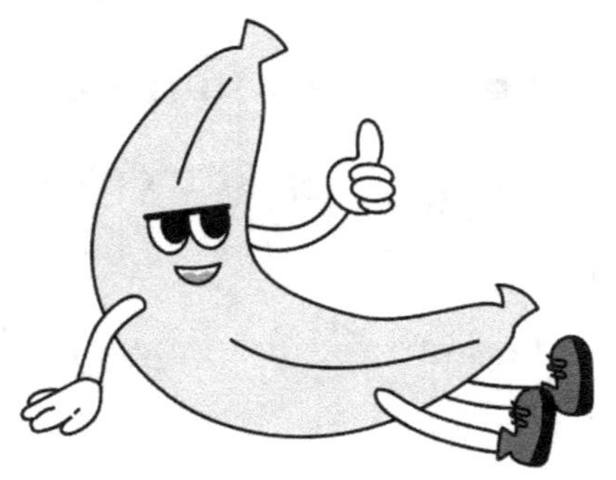

Chapter 3: The 7-Day Smoothie Challenge

Day 5: Orange Banana Smoothie:
A Burst of Refreshing Sweetness

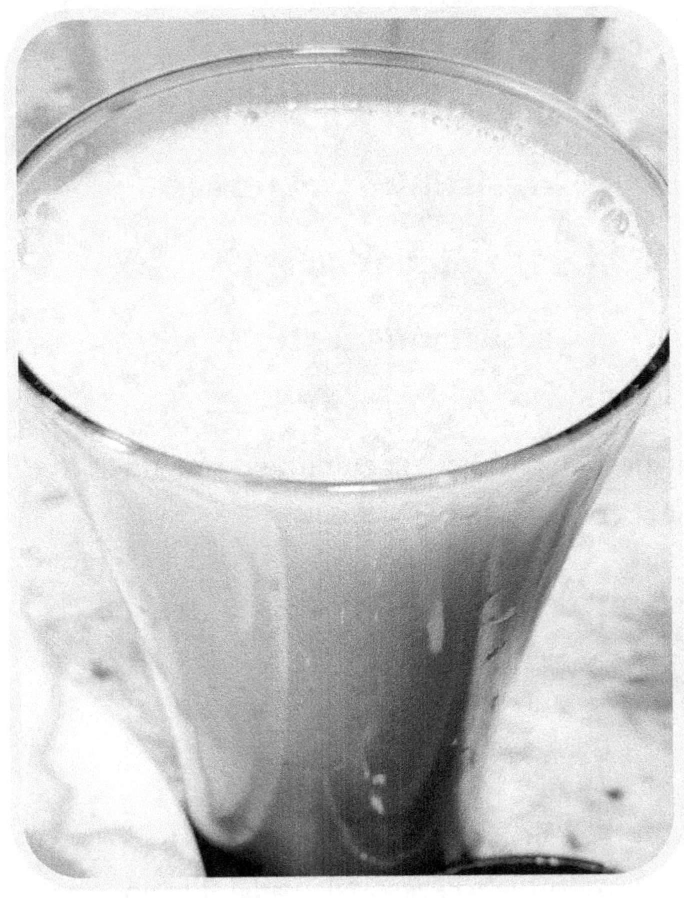

Stay tuned for Day 6 of our seven-day smoothie challenge, where we'll introduce another tantalizing recipe to keep your taste buds intrigued and your health journey on track. Don't forget to share your smoothie experiences and join our thriving community at www.modernlivingguide.com. Let's continue to inspire and support one another on this incredible path to continuous improvement!

Chapter 3: The 7-Day Smoothie Challenge

Day 6: Strawberry Banana Smoothie

Ah, the classic combination of strawberries and bananas. Today, we celebrate the timeless partnership of these two beloved fruits. Discover the:

Irresistible sweetness

Creaminess

Luscious texture

That emerges when strawberries and bananas unite in a blender. We'll guide you through various recipes using strawberries that are:

Fresh

Frozen

Dried

Allowing you to adapt your smoothie to seasonal availability and personal preference.

Chapter 3: The 7-Day Smoothie Challenge

Day 6: Strawberry Banana Smoothie

Welcome back to the world of smoothies, where a collision of:

Creativity

Freshness

Taste

Brings you delicious and nutritious concoctions. Get ready to embark on a flavor-packed journey with one of our all-time favorites: the Strawberry Banana Smoothie.

Smoothies offer a world of possibilities, allowing you to tailor your blend to match your:

Personal taste

Nutritional requirements

Health goals

Whether you prefer fruits, vegetables, or a combination of both, the power is in your hands. You have complete control over your smoothie adventure with:

Options for dairy or non-dairy milk

Inclusion of nuts or seeds

Plethora of other ingredients

Chapter 3: The 7-Day Smoothie Challenge

Day 6: Strawberry Banana Smoothie

We're excited to showcase the beauty of fruit smoothies. From banana smoothies to strawberry smoothies, the possibilities are endless. And what could be better than combining these two beloved fruits to create a symphony of flavors that will tantalize your taste buds? We've also explored exciting combinations like the:

Orange Banana Smoothie

Banana Spinach Smoothie

Banana Pear Smoothie

However, one combination stands out as a top favorite:

The timeless

Refreshing

Easy-to-make

Strawberry Banana Smoothie.

Chapter 3: The 7-Day Smoothie Challenge

Day 6: Strawberry Banana Smoothie:
A Perfect Blend of Refreshment and Delight

Welcome to Day 6 of our seven-day smoothie challenge! Today, we have a classic and beloved combination in store for you: the Strawberry Banana Smoothie. This timeless duo of strawberries and bananas creates a heavenly blend of:

Sweetness

Creaminess

Richness

That will leave you craving more. Let's dive into the recipe!

Ingredients:

1 cup or bowl of fresh or frozen strawberries

1 ripe banana

1 cup of almond milk. (Unsweetened)

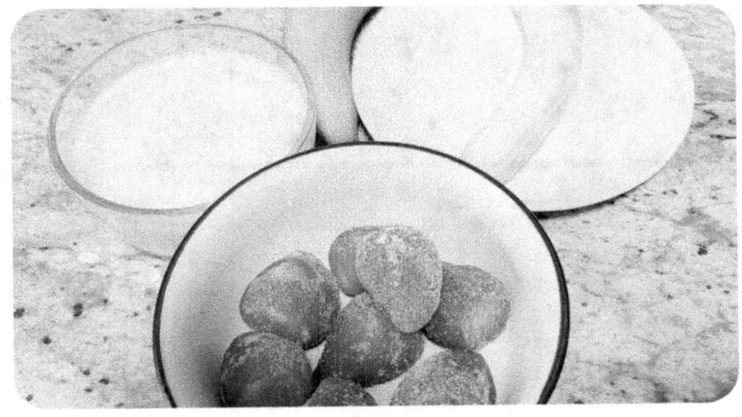

Chapter 3: The 7-Day Smoothie Challenge

Day 6: Strawberry Banana Smoothie:
A Perfect Blend of Refreshment and Delight

Instructions:

When utilizing fresh strawberries, remember to wash and remove the stems. If using frozen strawberries, no preparation is needed.

Peel the ripe banana. Cut it into smaller pieces.

Place the unsweetened almond milk into the blender.

Place the strawberries and banana into your blender.

Blend all the ingredients together. Blend at high speed until you reach a smooth and creamy texture.

Give the smoothie a taste and adjust the sweetness or thickness by adding more strawberries or almond milk if desired.

Pour the strawberry banana smoothie into a glass or jar, and consider garnishing with a fresh strawberry on top for an extra touch of elegance.

Take a moment to admire the beautiful blend of:

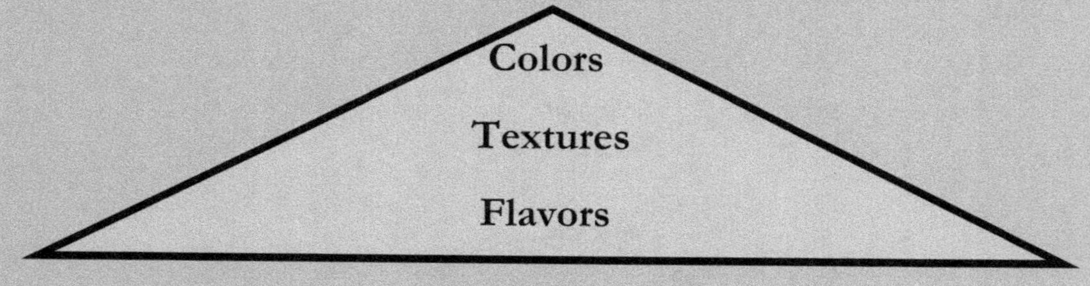

Before indulging in your luscious strawberry banana smoothie.

Chapter 3: The 7-Day Smoothie Challenge

Day 6: Strawberry Banana Smoothie:
A Perfect Blend of Refreshment and Delight

This smoothie is a timeless classic, combining:

The natural sweetness of strawberries
The smooth and creamy texture of bananas
The richness and nutty flavor of almond milk

The strawberries infuse the blend with their bright and juicy flavor, while the bananas contribute a velvety richness and an abundance of potassium.

Sip on this delightful concoction as a:

Refreshing breakfast option
Satisfying snack
Guilt-free dessert

With each sip, you'll experience the harmony of flavors and the nutritional benefits of these powerhouse fruits, including:

Fiber
Vitamins
Antioxidants

Whether you use fresh or frozen strawberries, this smoothie will transport you to a summer paradise and leave your taste buds dancing with joy.

Chapter 3: The 7-Day Smoothie Challenge

Day 6: Strawberry Banana Smoothie:
A Perfect Blend of Refreshment and Delight

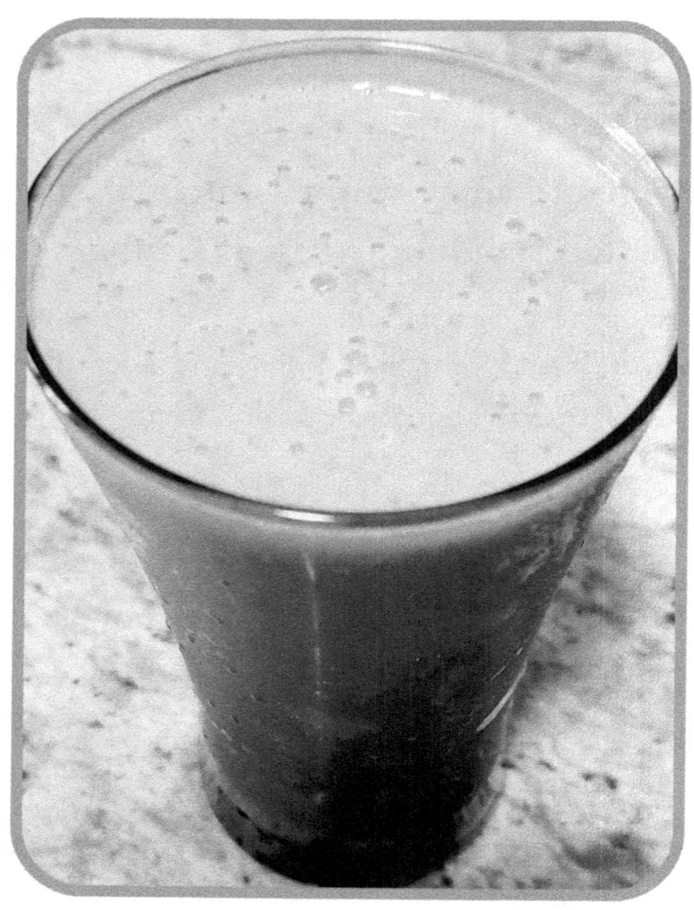

Stay tuned for Day 7, the final day of our seven-day smoothie challenge, where we'll introduce an exceptional smoothie to conclude our journey on a high note. Don't forget to share your smoothie experiences and join our thriving community at www.modernlivingguide.com. Let's continue to inspire and support one another on this incredible path to continuous improvement!

Chapter 3: The 7-Day Smoothie Challenge

Day 7: Strawberry Lemon Smoothie

We conclude our 7-day challenge with a burst of vibrant flavors. Immerse yourself in the tangy brightness of strawberries and the zesty freshness of lemon. Experience the:

Rejuvenating

Uplifting

Revitalizing

Properties of this invigorating blend. As we bid farewell to the challenge, we'll provide you with exciting variations like:

Adding mint leaves

A sprinkle of lemon zest

A drizzle of honey

Allowing you to savor every sip of this refreshing delight.

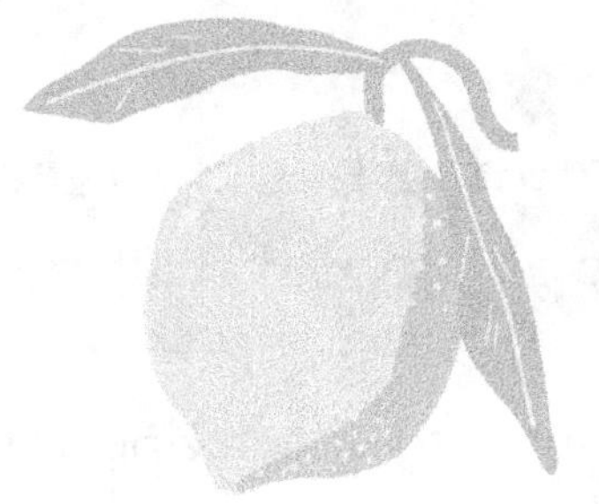

Chapter 3: The 7-Day Smoothie Challenge

Day 7: Strawberry Lemon Smoothie

Welcome back to our journey through the world of smoothies, where we celebrate the full spectrum of taste profiles. While we adore sweet flavors, we also appreciate the beauty of:

Bitterness
Sourness
Tanginess

In fact, a healthy balance of sweet and sour can add a delightful twist to our day. Not only that, but the sour taste is believed to stimulate the secretion of digestive enzymes, aiding in the process of digestion.

As we continue our exploration of healthy smoothie recipes, we dive deeper into the realm of fruit smoothies. By now, you're well aware that fruit smoothies can be:

Delicious
Filling
Nutritious

They also assist the body in:

Breaking down food more efficiently
Promoting better digestion
Supporting overall health

So, get ready for our latest addition to the recipe for fruit smoothies: the Strawberry Lemon Smoothie.

Chapter 3: The 7-Day Smoothie Challenge

Day 7: Strawberry Lemon Smoothie

Within the world of fruits, you'll find an array of options with profiles like:

Bitter
Sour
Tangy

From:

Cranberries and tamarind
Green mangoes and grapefruits
Passion fruit and pomegranate

The possibilities are endless. Even some sweet fruits, like:

Green apples
Green grapes
Green bananas

Can surprise us with their hint of tanginess. However, when we seek the ultimate sourness and tanginess, we turn to our beloved lemons and limes—they never disappoint.

We've created a perfect union of sweet and sour with our Strawberry Lemon Smoothie recipe.

The strawberries provide a mild to medium sweetness
The almond milk provides creaminess and nuttiness
The lemon brings that desired bitter, sour, and tangy taste to the mix

The combination results in a well-balanced blend of flavors that we thoroughly enjoyed, and we believe you will too.

Chapter 3: The 7-Day Smoothie Challenge

Day 7: Strawberry Lemon Smoothie: Embrace the Tangy Twist

Congratulations! You've made it to the final day of our seven-day smoothie challenge. Today, we have a delightful blend that combines the sweetness of strawberries with the zesty tang of lemons: the Strawberry Lemon Smoothie. Get ready to indulge in this invigorating and refreshing concoction. Let's dive into the recipe!

Ingredients:

1 cup or bowl of fresh or frozen strawberries

½ lemon

1 ripe banana (optional)

1 cup of almond milk. (Unsweetened)

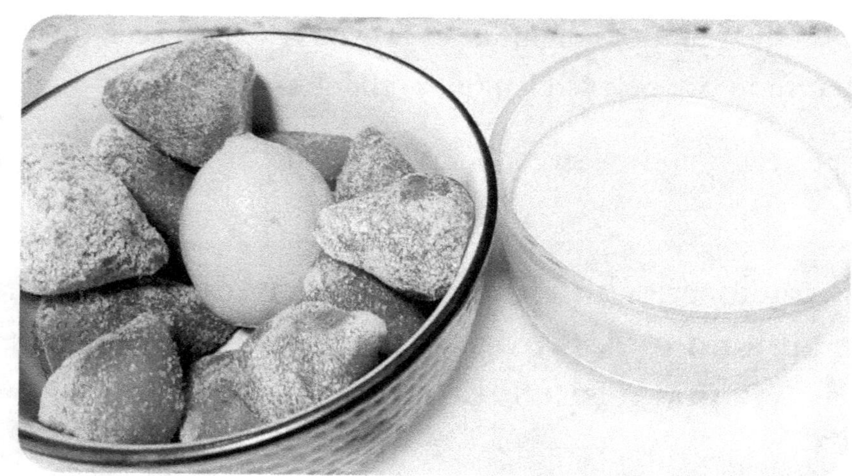

Chapter 3: The 7-Day Smoothie Challenge

Day 7: Strawberry Lemon Smoothie: Embrace the Tangy Twist

Instructions:

When utilizing fresh strawberries, remember to wash and remove the stems. If using frozen strawberries, no preparation is needed.

Squeeze the juice of ½ lemon, ensuring there are no seeds.

Peel the ripe banana. Cut it into smaller pieces. (Optional)

Place the unsweetened almond milk into the blender.

Place the strawberries, lemon juice, and banana into your blender.

Blend all the ingredients together. Blend at high speed until you reach a smooth and creamy texture.

Give the smoothie a taste and adjust the sweetness or tanginess by adding more strawberries or lemon juice if desired.

Pour the strawberry lemon smoothie into a glass or jar, and consider garnishing with a strawberry slice or a lemon wedge for an extra burst of visual appeal.

Take a moment to appreciate the vibrant colors and invigorating aroma before enjoying the last sip of your seven-day smoothie challenge.

Chapter 3: The 7-Day Smoothie Challenge

Day 7: Strawberry Lemon Smoothie: Embrace the Tangy Twist

This smoothie is a perfect blend of:

The sweet juiciness of strawberries

The creaminess of almond milk

The refreshing tartness of lemons

The combination creates a harmonious symphony of flavors that will awaken your taste buds and leave you feeling revitalized.

As you savor this final smoothie of the challenge, you're treating yourself to:

Antioxidants

A burst of vitamin C

A myriad of health benefits

In essence:

The strawberries contribute to heart health and support immune function

The lemons provide detoxifying properties and aid digestion

The almond milk provides essential nutrients and dose of healthy fats

Chapter 3: The 7-Day Smoothie Challenge

Day 7: Strawberry Lemon Smoothie: Embrace the Tangy Twist

Whether you're:

Kicking off your day with an energy boost
Indulging in a mid-day-pick-me-up
Winding down with a refreshing treat

The Strawberry Lemon Smoothie is the perfect way to celebrate your accomplishment and embark on a journey towards a healthier lifestyle.

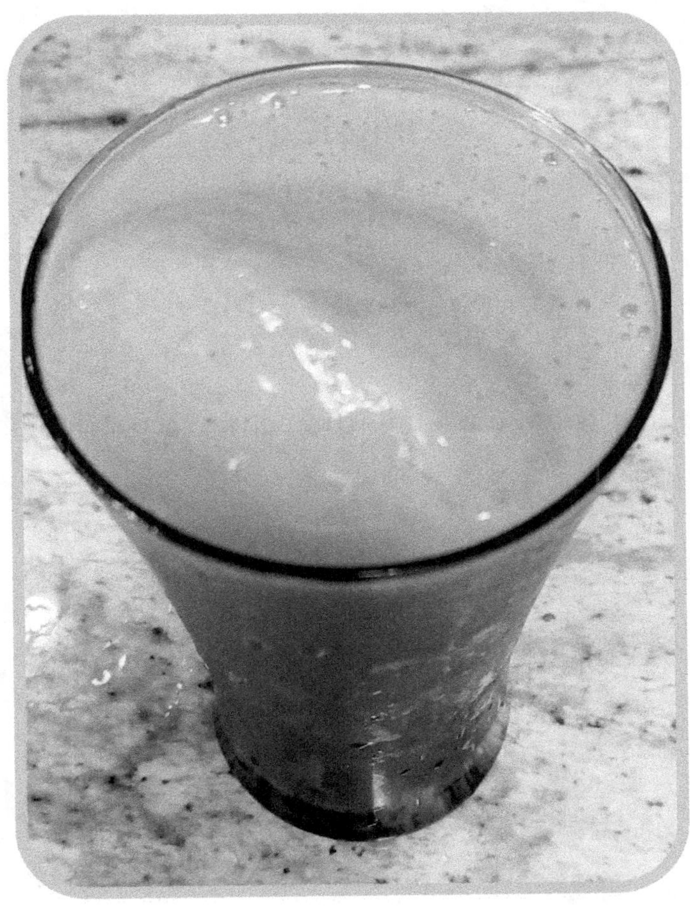

Chapter 3: The 7-Day Smoothie Challenge

Day 7: Strawberry Lemon Smoothie: Embrace the Tangy Twist

We hope you've enjoyed the seven-day smoothie challenge and discovered a newfound love for incorporating:

Nutritious

Nourishing

Delicious

Smoothies into your daily routine. Remember to share your experiences and join our thriving community at www.modernlivingguide.com, where we explore methods to enhance your:

Physical

Mental

Social

Spiritual health

Cheers to your health and continuous improvement! Keep blending and embracing the joy of living a vibrant life.

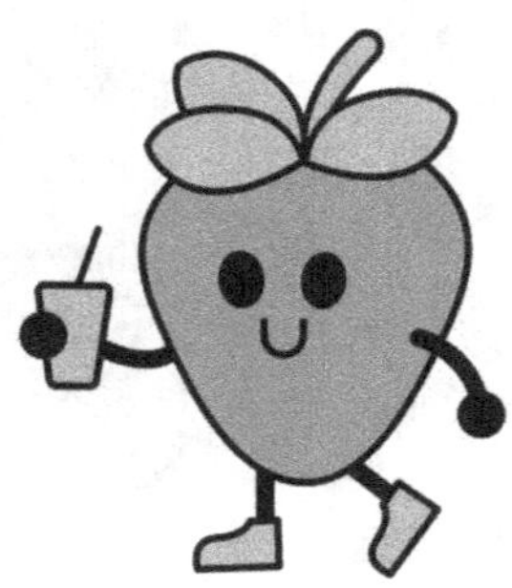

Conclusion:

Congratulations on completing "The 7-Day Smoothie Challenge: How to Unleash the Power of Everyday Smoothies!" You've embarked on a flavorful journey that has:

Transformed your mornings
Energized your day
Revitalized your body

Through this Book, you've discovered the joy of incorporating delicious and nutritious smoothies into your daily routine, and the impact has been truly remarkable.

Over the course of these seven days, you've explored a multitude of flavors, like:

The classic combinations of apples and bananas
The vibrant pairings of strawberries and lemons
The harmonious blend of banana and pear

Each smoothie has offered a unique experience:

Nourishing your body
Sustaining your energy
Tantalizing your taste buds

With a powerhouse of nutrients. You've awakened your creativity and learned to customize recipes to suit your preferences, making each blend a reflection of your own unique palate.

Conclusion:

Beyond the incredible taste sensations, you've witnessed firsthand the incredible benefits that everyday smoothies bring to your life:

You've experienced a surge of natural energy that sustains you throughout the day

Your nutrient intake has skyrocketed, ensuring your body receives the essential vitamins and minerals it needs to thrive

Your digestion has been supported, and your gut health has flourished

Weight management has become more possible, and you've found satisfaction in healthier choices

Your skin has become radiant, reflecting the nourishment within

Every sip has been a step towards a healthier, happier you.

But this is not the end of your smoothie journey. Armed with:

The knowledge
The skills
The inspiration

Gained from this challenge, you're now equipped to continue exploring the world of everyday smoothies. Let your creativity run wild as you experiment with new:

Ingredients
Combinations
Techniques

The possibilities are endless, and the rewards are limitless.

Conclusion:

Remember, smoothies are not just a fleeting trend; they are a lifestyle choice. They represent your:

Commitment to self-care
Dedication to nourishing your body
Desire to embrace the vibrant flavors nature has to offer

Make everyday smoothies a part of your ongoing journey towards optimal health and well-being.

As you bid farewell to "The 7-Day Smoothie Challenge," carry the knowledge and passion you've gained with you.

Blend
Sip
Savor

Your way to a vibrant and fulfilling life. Let every smoothie be a:

Celebration of your health
Testament to your vitality
Reminder of the power you have

To nurture yourself.

Conclusion:

Cheers to the wonderful world of everyday smoothies, and to the incredible transformation that awaits you as you continue this delicious and nutritious journey. Embrace:

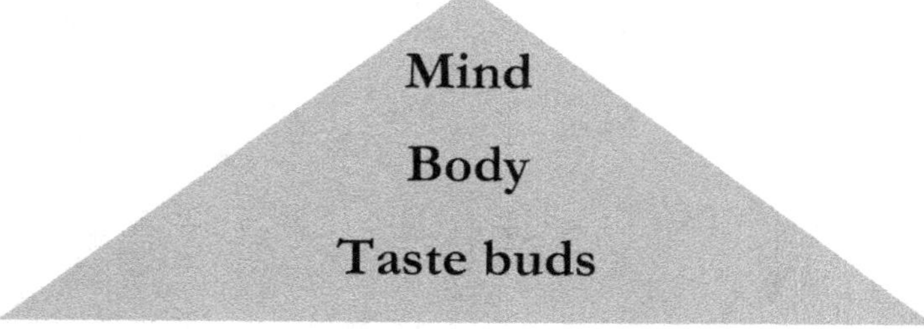

That comes from every sip. Get ready to experience the full potential of your:

Cheers to a vibrant and healthy life fueled by the power of everyday smoothies!

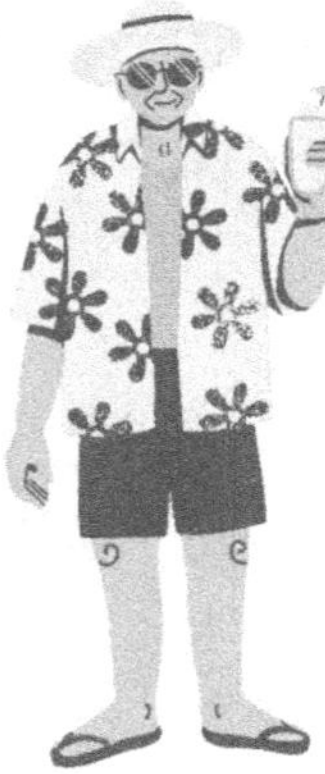

Chapter 4:
Your 7-Day Smoothie Challenge Journey Begins

Congratulations on reaching this exciting chapter of your smoothie adventure! By now:

You've learned about the wonderful world of everyday smoothies

Explored a variety of delectable recipes

Discovered the perfect balance of flavors to suit your taste buds

It's time to take the reins and create your own 7-day smoothie challenge!

Are you ready to embrace the challenge and embark on a week-long journey of:

Nourishment

Vitality

Delight

We're here to guide you through the process and provide you with a journal section where you can jot down your smoothie creations each day.

Chapter 4:
Your 7-Day Smoothie Challenge Journey Begins

Remember, the beauty of a smoothie challenge lies in its flexibility. You have the freedom to:

Choose your favorite fruits
Experiment with different combinations
Tailor the challenge to align with your personal health goals

Whether you're looking to:

Boost your energy
Incorporate more greens into your diet
Simply enjoy a daily dose of deliciousness

The smoothie challenge is the perfect opportunity to do so.

In the journal section provided, write down your 7-day smoothie challenge plan. Allow your imagination to roam freely as you visualize:

The flavors
The textures
The nutritional benefits

You want to experience each day. Will you start with a classic banana smoothie on day one, or perhaps venture into the world of green smoothies with a spinach and pineapple blend? The choice is yours.

Chapter 4:
Your 7-Day Smoothie Challenge Journey Begins
Day 1: Banana Berry Blast

As you repeat the challenge 7-days at a time, feel free to modify and adapt your recipes based on your preferences and the ingredients available to you. This is your personal journey, and it should reflect your unique tastes and desires.

To get you started, let's consider what your Day 1 smoothie challenge could look like:

Ingredients:

1 ripe banana

1 cup of mixed berries. Such as:

Strawberries

Blueberries

Raspberries

1 cup of almond milk. (unsweetened)

A small amount of spinach (if desired) to add an extra nutritional boost.

Chapter 4:
Your 7-Day Smoothie Challenge Journey Begins
Day 1: Banana Berry Blast

Instructions:

Remove the banana's peel and put it into the blender.

Add the mixed berries, allowing their vibrant flavors to mingle with the banana.

Pour in the almond milk, creating a smooth and creamy texture.

If you desire an additional nutritional boost, add a handful of spinach to the mix.

Blend the ingredients until they become perfectly combined and delightfully smooth.

Pour your banana berry blast into a glass, and let the journey begin!

As you savor each sip of this invigorating smoothie, take a moment to appreciate the:

Freshness of the berries

Smoothness of the almond milk

Creamy sweetness of the banana

Jot down your thoughts and observations in the journal section, noting the flavors that stood out to you and how the smoothie made you feel.

Chapter 4:
Your 7-Day Smoothie Challenge Journey Begins

Now, it's time for you to continue the challenge. Fill out the journal sections provided for the remaining six days, letting your creativity flow as you experiment with different:

Fruits

Flavors

Textures

Feel free to revisit some of the recipes we've shared throughout this Book or create entirely new combinations that excite your taste buds.

Remember, the 7-day smoothie challenge is just the beginning. You can repeat the challenge for as long as you desire, allowing yourself to continually explore new recipes and enjoy the benefits of these beverages that are:

Nourishing

Revitalizing

Delicious

Embrace the journey, and may every sip of your smoothie creations lead you towards a version of yourself that is more:

Healthier

Energized

Vibrant

We can't wait to hear about your smoothie challenge experience—share with us along the way your

Progress

Discoveries

Favorite recipes

Cheers to your 7-day smoothie challenge, and the exciting possibilities that lie ahead!

Chapter 5:
Join Our Thriving Community at Modern Living Guide

Congratulations on completing this journey through the world of everyday smoothies! You've:

Discovered a plethora of delicious recipes
Gained insights into the power of healthy ingredients
Created your own 7-day smoothie challenge

But our mission at Modern Living Guide extends far beyond smoothies alone.

Join our thriving community at www.modernlivingguide.com and start a transformative journey towards continuous improvement. At Modern Living Guide, we believe in nurturing all aspects of your well-being and health such as:

Physical

Mental

Social

Spiritual

On our platform, we discover various methods and practices to improve every part of your life.

As you've seen in this Book, just adding smoothies to your daily routine can greatly improve your overall health. But we're here to support you on a broader level, offering:

Guidance

Inspiration

Empowerment

Enabling you to prosper and excel in all facets of your life.

Chapter 5:
Join Our Thriving Community at Modern Living Guide

At Modern Living Guide, you'll find a wealth of resources, including:

Articles
Guides
Advice

Each element crafted to empower you on your path towards complete well-being:

From fitness and nutrition tips
To mindfulness practices and self-care techniques
To mental wellness and stress management

We cover a vast array of topics that will:

Inspire
Empower
Motivate

You to live a life that is more fulfilling and balanced.

By joining our community, you'll gain access to a supportive network of like-minded individuals who share a common goal: to live their best lives and inspire others to do the same.

Engage in discussions
Share your experiences
Connect with individuals

Who are on a similar path of personal growth and self-discovery.

Chapter 5:
Join Our Thriving Community at Modern Living Guide

So, take the next step towards unlocking your full potential and becoming the best version of yourself. Visit www.modernlivingguide.com and become a part of our thriving community. Together, we will:

Explore new possibilities

Learn from one another

Embark on a journey

Towards continuous improvement.

Thank you for joining us on this smoothie adventure, and we look forward to welcoming you to the Modern Living Guide community. Cheers to a life of vibrant health and boundless joy!

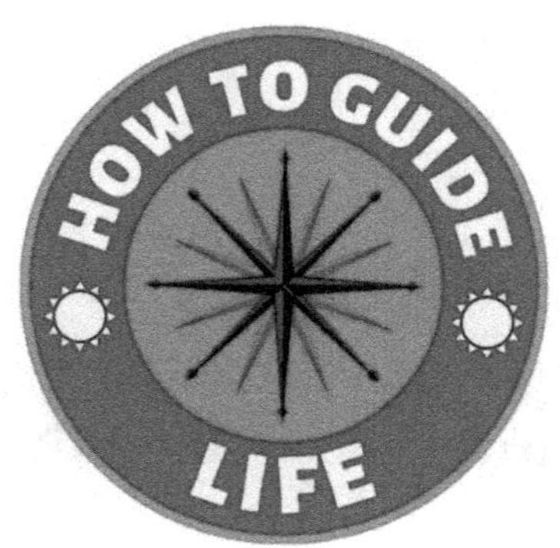

About the Author

Taylor Johnson is an enthusiastic advocate for healthy living and a passionate believer in the power of nourishing our bodies and minds. With experience in nutrition and a deep love for exploring creative ways to promote well-being, Taylor has dedicated her life to inspiring others to embrace a holistic approach to health.

Driven by a curiosity for discovering the best methods to enhance physical, mental, social, and spiritual well-being, Taylor has spent years studying and experimenting with various practices, blending the worlds of science and intuition to create a comprehensive guide for modern living.

As the author of this Book, Taylor's goal is to empower readers like you to take charge of your health and embark on a journey of continuous improvement. By sharing delicious smoothie recipes, practical tips, and insights into the benefits of everyday smoothies, Taylor aims to ignite your passion for wholesome nutrition and inspire you to make positive changes in your life.

With a deep understanding of the importance of balance, Taylor encourages a holistic approach to wellness, recognizing that true health encompasses not only physical vitality but also mental clarity, emotional well-being, and a strong sense of connection to oneself and others.

Beyond the pages of this Book, Taylor continues to explore new avenues for promoting a healthy and fulfilling lifestyle. As a wellness advocate, Taylor shares her knowledge and experiences through various platforms, including courses, and her thriving online community at Modern Living Guide.

Taylor's warm and relatable writing style invites you to join her on a journey towards a vibrant and joyful existence. Through her experiences and insights, she empowers readers to take small, meaningful steps towards achieving their health goals and unlocking their true potential.

About the Author

As you delve into the world of everyday smoothies and embrace the 7-day smoothie challenge, remember that Taylor is right there with you, cheering you on every step of the way. Through her words, she hopes to inspire and motivate you to live your best life— one delicious sip at a time.

So, grab your blender, gather your favorite ingredients, and get ready to embark on a transformative journey towards vibrant health and well-being. Let Taylor Johnson be your guide, empowering you to make positive choices and embrace a holistic approach to living. Cheers to a life of vitality, nourishment, and continuous growth!

Resources

Welcome to the Resources Section of " The 7-Day Smoothie Challenge: How to Unleash the Power of Everyday Smoothies!"! Here, you will find a collection of valuable tools and resources to enhance your smoothie journey and make it a truly enriching experience. We understand that creating and documenting your own smoothie recipes, tracking your progress, and staying organized are key elements to a successful and enjoyable smoothie challenge. That's why we have provided you with a Recipe Writing Section, a Journaling Section, and a 7-Day Calendar Section to support you every step of the way.

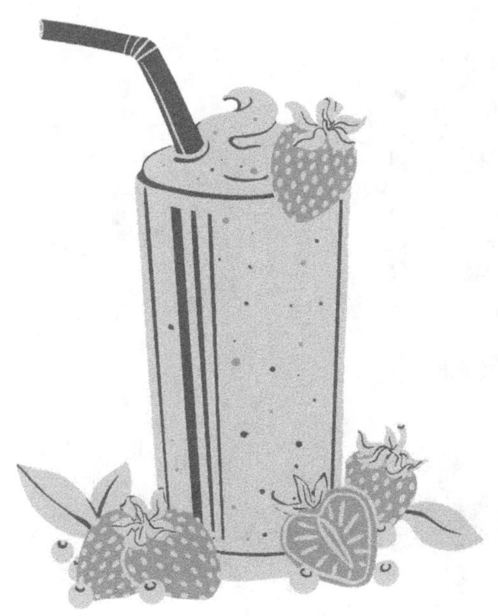

Smoothie Recipe: Your 7-Day Smoothie Challenge

Unleash your creativity and write down your own unique smoothie recipes in this dedicated section. We encourage you to experiment with different combinations of fruits, vegetables, liquids, and enhancements to create your personalized smoothie masterpieces. Use the recipe template provided to jot down the ingredients, measurements, and instructions for each creation. Feel free to make notes on the taste, texture, and any modifications you made. This section will become your personal smoothie recipe collection, allowing you to revisit and recreate your favorites time and time again.

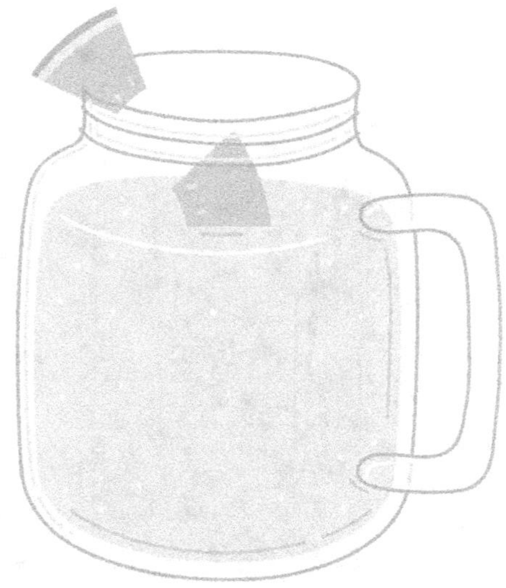

Smoothie Recipe: Your 7-Day Smoothie Challenge

Welcome to your smoothie recipe journal! Use this section to record your favorite smoothie recipes, experiment with new flavor combinations, and document your experience during your 7-day smoothie challenge. Get ready to blend, sip, and enjoy the journey to a healthier you!

Day 1: ____

Smoothie Recipe:

____

____

____

____

____

Ingredients:

____

____

____

____

____

____

Smoothie Recipe: Your 7-Day Smoothie Challenge

Day 1: ___________________________________

Instructions:

____

____

____

____

____

____

____

____

____

____

Taste and Texture Notes:

____

____

Overall Experience:

____

____

____

Smoothie Recipe: Your 7-Day Smoothie Challenge

Day 2: _______________________________

____

____

____

Smoothie Recipe:

____

____

____

____

____

____

Ingredients:

____

____

____

____

____

____

Smoothie Recipe: Your 7-Day Smoothie Challenge

Day 2: _______________________________________

____

____

Instructions:

____

____

____

____

____

____

____

____

____

Taste and Texture Notes:

____

____

Overall Experience:

____

____

Smoothie Recipe: Your 7-Day Smoothie Challenge

Day 3: _______________________________________

____

____

____

Smoothie Recipe:

____

____

____

____

____

____

Ingredients:

____

____

____

____

____

____

Smoothie Recipe: Your 7-Day Smoothie Challenge

Day 3: ____

____

____

Instructions:

____

____

____

____

____

____

____

____

____

Taste and Texture Notes:

____

____

Overall Experience:

____

____

____

Smoothie Recipe: Your 7-Day Smoothie Challenge

Day 4: _______________________________________

____

____

____

Smoothie Recipe:

____

____

____

____

____

____

Ingredients:

____

____

____

____

____

____

____

Smoothie Recipe: Your 7-Day Smoothie Challenge

Day 4: _______________________________________

____

____

Instructions:

____

____

____

____

____

____

____

____

Taste and Texture Notes:

____

____

Overall Experience:

____

____

____

Smoothie Recipe: Your 7-Day Smoothie Challenge

Day 5: _______________________________________

____

____

____

Smoothie Recipe:

____

____

____

____

____

____

Ingredients:

____

____

____

____

____

Smoothie Recipe: Your 7-Day Smoothie Challenge

Day 5: _______________________________________

____

____

Instructions:

____

____

____

____

____

____

____

____

Taste and Texture Notes:

____

____

Overall Experience:

____

____

____

Smoothie Recipe: Your 7-Day Smoothie Challenge

Day 6: _______________________________________

____

____

____

Smoothie Recipe:

____

____

____

____

____

____

Ingredients:

____

____

____

____

____

____

____

Smoothie Recipe: Your 7-Day Smoothie Challenge

Day 6: _______________________________________

____

____

Instructions:

____

____

____

____

____

____

____

____

Taste and Texture Notes:

____

____

Overall Experience:

____

____

____

Smoothie Recipe: Your 7-Day Smoothie Challenge

Day 7: ______________________________________

____

____

____

Smoothie Recipe:

____

____

____

____

____

____

____

Ingredients:

____

____

____

____

____

____

____

Smoothie Recipe: Your 7-Day Smoothie Challenge

Day 7: _______________________________________

____

____

Instructions:

____

____

____

____

____

____

____

____

Taste and Texture Notes:

____

____

Overall Experience:

____

____

____

Smoothie Recipe: Your 7-Day Smoothie Challenge

Additional Notes:

Use this space to jot down any additional smoothie recipe ideas, flavor variations, or ingredient substitutions that you would like to try in the future. This is your opportunity to get creative and continue exploring the world of delicious smoothies. Have fun and keep blending!

Reflections:

Reflect on your 7-day smoothie challenge experience. How did incorporating smoothies into your daily routine make you feel? Did you notice any positive changes in your energy levels, digestion, or overall well-being? Take a moment to celebrate your achievements and set new goals for your continued smoothie journey.

Remember to listen to your body, adjust recipes to suit your taste preferences, and have fun with the process. Cheers to a vibrant and delicious smoothie challenge!

Note: This smoothie recipe journal is designed to help you document your own smoothie creations. Feel free to use the provided spaces to write down your favorite recipes, ingredient quantities, and personal notes. Happy blending!

Additional Notes:

____

____

____

____

____

____

Smoothie Recipe: Your 7-Day Smoothie Challenge

Additional Notes:

Smoothie Recipe: Your 7-Day Smoothie Challenge

Additional Notes:

Self-Journaling: Your 7-Day Smoothie Challenge

Congratulations on taking the first step towards a healthier and more vibrant lifestyle with " The 7-Day Smoothie Challenge: How to Unleash the Power of Everyday Smoothies!" Book. Now, it's time to embark on your own 7-day smoothie challenge and discover the transformative power of incorporating these nutritious blends into your daily routine. This self-journaling section is designed to help you track your progress, reflect on your experience, and make the most out of your smoothie journey. Grab a pen and let's get started!

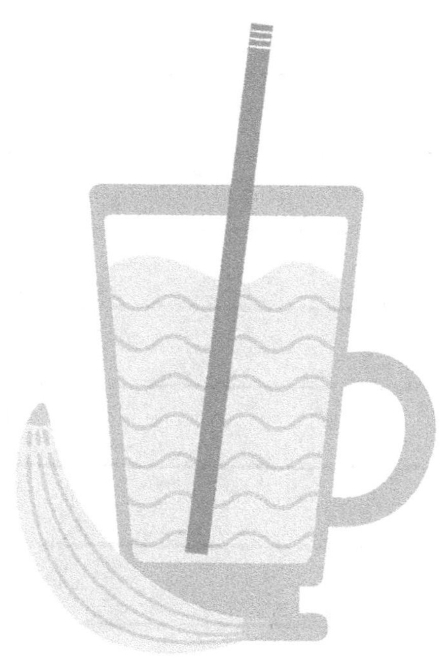

Self-Journaling: Your 7-Day Smoothie Challenge

Welcome to your 7-day smoothie challenge! Prepare yourself for an enriching voyage towards improved well-being and energy levels. Use this self-journaling section to document your experience, track your progress, and reflect on the positive changes that each day brings. Let's dive in and make the most out of your smoothie challenge!

Day 1: ____

Today marks the beginning of your smoothie challenge. Describe the smoothie you made and the ingredients you used. Take note of how it tastes and any immediate effects you notice. How does it make you feel? Are you excited to kickstart your journey towards a healthier lifestyle?

____

____

____

____

____

____

____

____

____

____

____

Self-Journaling: Your 7-Day Smoothie Challenge

Day 2: ____

Share your experience with today's smoothie. Did you try any new flavor combinations or ingredients? How did it contribute to your energy levels and overall well-being? Take a moment to contemplate the obstacles you encountered and the strategies you employed to conquer them. Remember, each day is an opportunity for growth and exploration.

Self-Journaling: Your 7-Day Smoothie Challenge

Day 3: ____

Document today's smoothie adventure. Did you experiment with different textures or ingredients? How did it impact your digestion and satiety levels? Take a moment to reflect on the positive changes you've experienced so far and the potential long-term benefits of incorporating smoothies into your daily routine.

Self-Journaling: Your 7-Day Smoothie Challenge

Day 4: _______________________________

Describe the smoothie you enjoyed today and how it fueled your body. Did you notice any changes in your energy levels or mood throughout the day? Reflect on the role of smoothies in supporting your overall well-being and promoting a healthy lifestyle. Celebrate your dedication to prioritizing self-care.

Self-Journaling: Your 7-Day Smoothie Challenge

Day 5: ____

Share your thoughts on today's smoothie creation. How did it contribute to your hydration levels and refreshment? Did you try any new liquid bases or flavor combinations? Take a moment to reflect on the importance of staying adequately hydrated and how smoothies can help you achieve that goal.

Self-Journaling: Your 7-Day Smoothie Challenge

Day 6: _______________________________

Describe the smoothie you made today and how it satisfied your taste buds. Did you experiment with any unique ingredients or superfoods? Reflect on the joy of discovering new flavors and nourishing your body with a variety of fruits and vegetables. Embrace the adventure of your smoothie challenge.

Self-Journaling: Your 7-Day Smoothie Challenge

Day 7: ____

Congratulations on completing your 7-day smoothie challenge! Share your overall experience and reflections. How have the smoothies impacted your energy levels, mood, and overall well-being? Reflect on the positive changes you've witnessed and how you plan to incorporate smoothies into your future routine.

Self-Journaling: Your 7-Day Smoothie Challenge

Additional Reflections:

Use this space to jot down any additional reflections, insights, or lessons learned throughout your 7-day smoothie challenge. Celebrate your successes, acknowledge any obstacles you overcame, and set new goals for your continued smoothie journey. Remember, this is just the beginning of a lifelong commitment to nourishing your body and embracing a healthier lifestyle.

Keep blending, keep journaling, and embrace the deliciousness and health benefits of smoothies! Enjoy the process, savor each sip, and take pride in the positive choices you're making. Get ready to experience the transformative power of smoothies in your life.

Cheers to a healthier, more vibrant you!

Additional Reflections:

____

____

____

____

____

____

____

____

Self-Journaling: Your 7-Day Smoothie Challenge

Additional Reflections:

Self-Journaling: Your 7-Day Smoothie Challenge

Additional Reflections:

7-Day Smoothie Calendar

Congratulations on embarking on your 7-day smoothie challenge! Use this calendar to plan and track your daily smoothie creations. As you sip your way through the week, mark off each day to celebrate your progress. Prepare yourself for a week filled with delectable and nourishing smoothies!

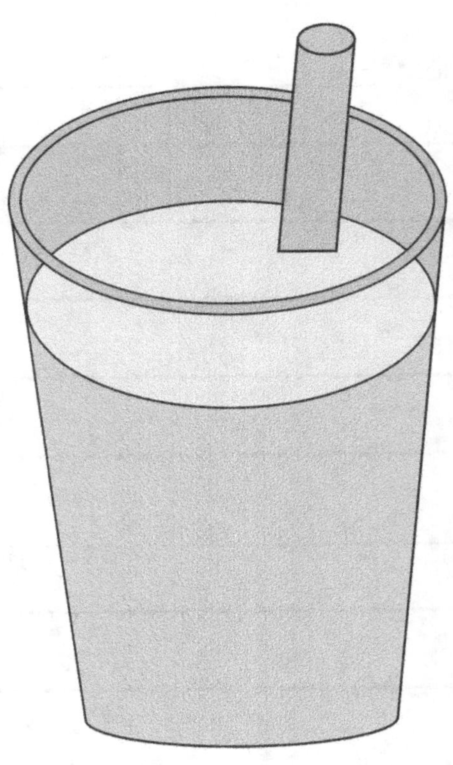

7-Day Smoothie Calendar

Day 1: _______________________________________

____

Smoothie Recipe: _________________________________

____

____

____

____

Description/Taste Notes: ____________________________

____

____

____

____

Notes/Reflection: _________________________________

____

____

____

____

____

7-Day Smoothie Calendar

Day 2: ______________________________________

____

Smoothie Recipe: ________________________________

____

____

____

____

____

Description/Taste Notes: ________________________

____

____

____

____

____

Notes/Reflection: _______________________________

____

____

____

____

____

____

7-Day Smoothie Calendar

Day 3: _______________________________

____

Smoothie Recipe: _______________________________

____

____

____

____

Description/Taste Notes: _______________________________

____

____

____

____

____

Notes/Reflection: _______________________________

____

____

____

____

____

7-Day Smoothie Calendar

Day 4: _______________________________

____

Smoothie Recipe: _______________________________

____

____

____

____

____

Description/Taste Notes: _______________________________

____

____

____

____

Notes/Reflection: _______________________________

____

____

____

____

____

7-Day Smoothie Calendar

Day 5: _______________________________________

____

Smoothie Recipe: _______________________________

____

____

____

____

Description/Taste Notes: _______________________

____

____

____

____

Notes/Reflection: _______________________________

____

____

____

____

7-Day Smoothie Calendar

Day 6: _______________________________

____

Smoothie Recipe: ___________________________

____

____

____

____

Description/Taste Notes: _______________

____

____

____

____

Notes/Reflection: ___________________________

____

____

____

____

____

7-Day Smoothie Calendar

Day 7: _______________________________

____

Smoothie Recipe: _____________________

____

____

____

____

Description/Taste Notes: _______________

____

____

____

____

Notes/Reflection: ____________________

____

____

____

____

____

7-Day Smoothie Calendar

Notes and Reflections:

Use this space to jot down any additional notes, reflections, or adjustments you made to the recipes. Did you discover any new flavor combinations? How did the smoothies make you feel? Take a moment to reflect on your journey and celebrate your achievements.

Remember to listen to your body, adjust recipes to suit your taste preferences, and have fun experimenting with different ingredients. Enjoy your 7-day smoothie challenge and savor the goodness in every sip!

Note: This smoothie calendar is designed to help you plan and track your 7-day smoothie challenge. Feel free to use the provided spaces to write down your favorite recipes, taste notes, and personal reflections. Cheers to a week of nourishing and delicious smoothies!

Notes and Reflections:

____

____

____

____

____

____

____

____

____

7-Day Smoothie Calendar

Notes and Reflections:

____

____

____

____

____

____

____

____

____

____

____

____

____

____

7-Day Smoothie Calendar

Notes and Reflections: